SYMPTOM MANAGEMENT
IN
MULTIPLE SCLEROSIS

SYMPTOM MANAGEMENT IN MULTIPLE SCLEROSIS

Randall T. Schapiro, M.D.
Director of Rehabilitation and the Multiple Sclerosis Center
Fairview Hospital

and

Clinical Professor of Neurology, University of Minnesota
Minneapolis, Minnesota

Demos Publications
New York

Demos Publications   156 Fifth Avenue, New York, NY 10010

Made in the United States of America

Main entry under title: Symptom Management in Multiple Sclerosis

Library of Congress Cataloging in Publication Data: 86-72100
ISBN: 0-939957-02-7

DEDICATION

To our patients.

PREFACE

All too often people with multiple sclerosis are told there is little that can be done for their disease. In fact, however, the appropriate management of MS includes a variety of rehabilitative, medical, and psychological approaches. Management strategies fall into two general categories, those used to treat the underlying disease process, and those used to minimize and control specific symptoms, such as spasticity, bowel or bladder problems, or fatigue.

This volume focuses on the management of specific symptoms that may develop as the result of the disease process in multiple sclerosis. It is based on the management program developed at the Fairview Multiple Sclerosis Center in Minneapolis. For each type of problem encountered, appropriate rehabilitative therapies and medication are considered.

It is hoped that this book will be of assistance to the multiple sclerosis person and to his/her family and friends, as well as to health care professionals in the many fields that impinge upon MS management.

CONTENTS

CONTRIBUTORS

Julie Arndt, R.P.T.
Brenda Brelje, R.N.
Andre DeLoya, R.P.T., M.S.
Kathy J. Harowski, Ph.D.
Lisa Harris, O.T.R.
Mary Hooley, M.A.
Mary Lenling, O.T.R.
Jackie Metelak, O.T.R.
Esther Motyka, B.S., R.D.
Elizabeth Nager, M.S.W.
Cindy Phair, B.S.N., M.A.
Richard Werner, M.D.

ACKNOWLEDGMENTS

A medical team specializing in multiple sclerosis requires a large amount of teamwork. This book represents the teamwork of the Fairview Multiple Sclerosis Center, and many people participated in its development. All of the contributors (listed with each chapter) wish to acknowledge those who worked, inspired, and were invaluable to the culmination of this effort, including Esther Bearden, Clark Christianson, Tom Dennis, Mark Enger, Richard Howard, Kurt Metzner, William Miller, Judy Morgan, Ralph Ohrn, Dawn Schapiro, Pamela Tibbetts, and Janet Whiteford, and to Dr. Diana M. Schneider of Demos Publications.

Symptom Management in Multiple Sclerosis.
Randall T. Schapiro, M.D.;
© 1987 Demos Publications, New York.

MULTIPLE SCLEROSIS IS...

Multiple sclerosis (MS) is one of a broad category of **demyelinating** diseases, affecting the central nervous system (CNS)—the brain and spinal cord. **Myelin** is a fatty material that insulates nerves, acting much like the covering of an electric wire and allowing the nerve to transmit its impulses rapidly. It is the speed at which these impulses are conducted that permits smooth, rapid, and coordinated movements, performed with little conscious effort. In multiple sclerosis, the loss of myelin is accompanied by a loss of the ability to perform these movements. The sites where myelin is lost appear as hardened sclerotic (scar) areas, and because there tends to be many such areas within the nervous system, the term multiple sclerosis (literally, many scars) seems appropriate.

A WORD ABOUT ANATOMY...

Frequently throughout this book mention is made of the anatomy of the nerves and muscles. It is hoped that an overview here will provide quick reference for the reader. Additional, more specific information is included with each topic as needed.

There are really three fairly distinct "nervous systems" in the human body (Figure 1). The **central nervous system** (CNS) lies centrally in the body and has two major parts, the brain and spinal cord, which in turn have several subdivisions, each with its own unique role in regulating the body's functions.

The portion of the brain referred to as the **cerebrum** acts as a master control system, and is responsible for initiating all thought and movement. Memory, personality, vision, hearing, touch, and muscle tone are also housed within the cerebrum. Behind the cerebrum sits the **cerebellum**, which coordinates movement and "smooths" muscle activity. It permits balance when walking and the smooth use of hands and arms.

Beneath the cerebrum and cerebellum is the **brainstem**. It contains the nerves that control the eyes as well as the vital centers that are involved in breathing, heart rate, etc. Coming directly from the brainstem is the **spinal cord**, which functions very much like a large electric cord carrying messages from the brain centers above to and from the targets (parts of the body) below.

While numerous biochemical reactions occur in the brain and spinal cord, their major effect is to produce electrical activity that stimulates and regulates the parts of the body. This electricity is brought to the target structures very efficiently and effectively, with little loss from top to bottom. This can be accomplished so well because the entire system is well insulated and shielded by a fatty substance called **myelin**, which surrounds the conducting systems and allows the electrical nervous impulses to literally skip down the line with little loss. The myelin in the brain and spinal cord is produced by a specific type of cell called an **oligodendrocyte** (oligo). Both the oligo and the myelin appear to be injured in MS. The oligos disappear as the myelin that is affected becomes hardened and scarred, forming what is called a **plaque**, and causing a short-circuiting of electrical transmission.

The second nervous system connects the spinal cord to the arms and legs, and is responsible for transmitting the electrical messages to targeted muscles. It is called the **peripheral nervous system** (PNS). This system also contains myelin, although it is made by a different cell type than the oligo, one which does not appear to be affected in multiple sclerosis. Thus, while it is not uncommon to find leg or arm weakness in MS, the problem lies in the central conduction system (the brain and

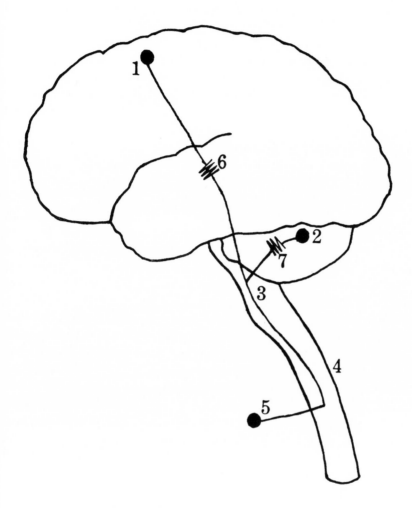

Figure 1. CNS pathway controlling arm movement. (1) The thought of raising the arm initiates the process by transmitting an electrical impulse. (2) Inputs from the cerebellum "smooth" the movement, allowing it to proceed in coordinated fashion. (3) The electrical impulse is conducted through the brainstem into the spinal cord. (4) The cord in turn conducts to the nerves that control the arm. (5) From the cord, the impulse goes through the nerves of the arm to the muscles, causing it to move as directed by the CNS. An interruption ("short-circuit") anywhere in this pathway will affect the strength or coordination of the movement. For example, a lesion at (6) will decrease the strength of the transmission, while one at (7) will decrease the ability to control movement in a coordinated fashion.

spinal cord) and not in the peripheral nerves leading out of the spinal cord.

The third nervous system is the **autonomic nervous system**. It has two divisions, the **sympathetic** and the **parasympathetic**. These are responsible for automatic types of function, e.g. heart beating, stomach growling, sweating, etc. This system also contains myelin, but like the PNS it is not directly affected by MS.

All of these nervous systems talk to each other. Thus, while only the CNS "gets" MS, the disease does produce indirect effects on the others and their functions.

SYMPTOMS OF MULTIPLE SCLEROSIS

Characteristics of MS include: 1) the onset of the disease is most common between the ages of 15 and 45; 2) remissions and exacerbations (improvements and flareups) are the rule, and 3) scattered areas in the central nervous system are diseased.

Because different areas of the brain and spinal cord are responsible for different kinds of movements and sensations, the neurologic deficit that results from an area of scarring is dependent on the exact location of the abnormality (lesion). For example, when an area of demyelination occurs in the area of the brain that is responsible for making coordinated movements (the cerebellum), such coordination becomes difficult. Because of this dependence of symptoms on the area of scarring, no two cases of MS are exactly alike, and symptoms vary considerably from one individual to another. In one person, the extent of the MS symptoms might be mild disturbances of gait and vision, whereas another might suffer a severe or complete sensory and motor loss.

While a number of persons with the disease are severely affected and become confined to wheelchairs, this is by no means the rule. Studies on large numbers of MS persons have shown that the majority live fairly normal lives with only minor incapacities, and some may have only one or two attacks of neurologic deficit.

A period during which new symptoms appear or existing ones increase in severity is termed an **exacerbation**, while the decrease of symptoms or a levelling off in their severity is a **remission**.

A specific characteristic of the disease is the presence of clinical symptoms that affect several sensory (touch, heat, cold) or motor (movement) functions in the CNS (brain and spinal cord), reflecting the existence of multiple sites of damage. Symptoms may fluctuate, or they may steadily progress in severity. Many patients have periods of stability lasting many years, and even those who ultimately progress to severe disability have long periods of more moderate symptoms.

While no predictions can be made as to the final degree of disability for an individual patient, the overall statistics should lead the MS person to have every reason for optimism.

POSSIBLE CAUSES OF MULTIPLE SCLEROSIS

While a specific cause of MS has not yet been determined, several theories seem plausible. MS is now generally considered an "auto-immune disease", one in which the body's own immune system, normally responsible for defending the body against viral and bacterial disease, begins for unknown reasons to attack normal body tissue, in this case the cells that make myelin. Susceptibility to autoimmune diseases appears to be at least in part genetic, so that while MS itself is not an hereditary disease, there may be an hereditary factor at work in making an individual susceptible to the development of the disease.

Additionally, while no virus has been consistently isolated in MS patients, many believe that a virus is originally responsible for "turning on" the immune system and making it behave in this abnormal fashion. Because of this, much research is devoted to looking for a virus "inducer" of MS. This search is further stimulated by the fact that environmental factors appear to be involved in the disease. People who spend the first 15 years or so of life in areas away from the equator have a much higher risk of developing the disease than do those who spend this period closer to the equator.

Research on MS has focused on several aspects of the disease. While it is hoped that once the cause (or, more probably, causes) of the disease has been found it will be possible to effect a cure or to prevent the disease from developing, in the meantime extensive research is ongoing into ways to manage the progress of the disease and specific symptoms as they develop. It is in these areas that progress has steadily been occurring, and it is possible for most MS individuals to live creative, meaningful and enjoyable lives.

Symptom Management in Multiple Sclerosis.
Randall T. Schapiro, M.D.;
© 1987 Demos Publications, New York.

THE MANAGEMENT OF MULTIPLE SCLEROSIS

Management strategies utilized to treat MS can be considered to fall into two general categories, those that are used to treat the underlying disease itself by shortening exacerbations and slowing the progress of the disease, and those that are used to minimize and control specific symptoms, such as spasticity, bowel and bladder problems, or fatigue.

Some general principles have been developed toward managing the disease, including minimizing over-fatigue, emotional stress and increases in body temperature, all of which can magnify symptoms.

Acute attacks are generally treated with corticosteroids (ACTH, Prednisone, Medrol, Decadron), which appear to shorten the exacerbation, in part by reducing the amount of swelling in areas of demyelination. A short course of therapy lasting one week to one month is initiated at the onset of a sudden attack, followed by a rapid tapering off over a defined period of time. When given in this manner, many of the side effects produced by the corticosteroids (including degeneration of the bones, cataracts, ulcers, obesity, decreased ability of the body to combat infections, salt and water balance problems) are kept to a minimum. The goal is to decrease swelling within the CNS, thus allowing unaffected nerves to function normally.

MS may involve a defect in the way the immune system "sees" myelin, so that it reacts to myelin as if it were a foreign tissue. Thus much of the focus of general management of the disease involves decreasing the activity of the immune system. Corticosteroids work, in part, through an effect on this system. Other drugs which also depress the activity of the immune system without the serious side effects of the corticosteroids are now being used in the long term management of MS. These include a series of drugs first used to treat cancer, which also involves a defect in the immune system. Imuran (azathiaprine) or Cytoxan (cyclophospha-mide) are examples of these. Their use in certain selected patients may allow for a slowing of the progression of some kinds of MS.

In addition to these very general treatments, a variety of therapies are available to treat the specific symptoms that can occur during the course of the disease. The remainder of this book is organized around such specific problem areas. It is designed to be read and used by the MS individual and his/her family and friends if and when specific symptoms develop. By no means do all or even many of these difficulties occur in all individuals. Virtually all of them, however, do have aggressive manage-ment strategies that can be utilized to minimize discomfort and incon-venience, especialy if begun when such symptoms first appear. It is hoped that this volume will assist the MS individual both to understand the problems that may result from his/her disease, and to work with the physician and other health care professionals in a manner optimally consistent with the best possible outcome of the disease.

The remainder of this volume is organized by symptom, beginning with the interrelated problems of spasticity, tremor, weakness, fatigue, and walking difficulties. These are among the most common, and most troublesome, problems encountered with MS. Their management is discussed in progressive fashion, beginning with a description of some of the simpler ways to control these symptoms, and progressing to more extreme measures that are occasionally needed when the problem is unusually severe.

This is followed by chapters on diet and exercise, since a sound nutrition and exercise program can lessen the impact of many of the symptoms of MS, especially those discussed in the initial chapters.

The remaining chapters address bladder and bowel problems, which are frequently encountered in MS, issues of sexuality, and a group of less serious but no less annoying symptoms that are commonly encountered. The final chapter, Adapting to MS, discusses issues that affect ones psychological adaptation to living with a disability, since many of the symptoms encountered in MS assume their rightful proportion when a good adjustment is made to living with the disease.

Symptom Management in Multiple Sclerosis.
Randall T. Schapiro, M.D.;
© 1987 Demos Publications, New York.

SPASTICITY

Andre DeLoya, R.P.T., M.S.
Julie Arndt, R.P.T.
Randall T. Schapiro, M.D.

In the normal nervous system, muscle groups work together such that when one contracts its opposing muscle relaxes. This coordination of movements makes them smooth and strong. In MS, this system of balance can be disturbed so that opposing muscles contract and relax at the same time, producing **spasticity**.

Spasticity tends to occur most frequently in a specific group of muscles that are responsible for maintaining our upright posture, referred to as anti-gravity or postural muscles. These include the muscles of the calf (gastrocnemius), thigh (quadriceps), buttock (gluteus maximus), groin (adductor) and occasionally the back (erector spinae).

When spasticity is present, the increased stiffness in the muscles means that a great deal of energy is required to perform everyday activities. Reducing the spasticity produces greater freedom of movement and strength, frequently accompanied by less fatigue and in-

11

creased coordination. The major ways by which spasticity is reduced include stretching exercises, physical therapy, and the use of drugs.

Physical Therapy

An appendix to the volume is included detailing a basic stretching program, as described in the exercises below.

The simplest and often most effective way of reducing spasticity is **passive stretching**, in which each affected joint is slowly moved into a position that stretches the spastic muscles. Once each muscle reaches its stretched position, it is held there for about a minute to allow it to slowly relax and release the undesired tension. This stretching program begins at the ankle, to stretch the calf muscle, then procedes upwards to the muscles in the back of the thigh, the buttocks, the groin, and, after turning from back to stomach, the muscles on the front of the thigh.

A key point is that some generalized relaxation of all spastic muscles can be obtained by first stretching the muscles of the calf. An ankle tilt board as shown in Figure 1 can be used for this purpose; the patient stands on the board with his back comfortably against a wall.

Independent Stretching

An independent stretching program based on some of the same principles used in physical therapy can be used at home. A tilt board as described above can be built of plywood, and tilted to an angle suggested by a therapist, or which has been found by experimenting to be most effective. Standing on the board for two or three minutes stretches the calf muscles, and some generalized relaxation will spread throughout other spastic muscles. The tilt board is best used to "boost" the relaxation achieved by a thorough stretching program performed early each morning.

A **thorough stretching program** consists of a series of exercises performed in specific sitting or lying positions that allow gravity to aid in stretching specific muscles. While in the sitting position, a towel or long belt may be used to pull on the forefoot and ankle to stretch the calf, or to stretch the thigh muscles when lying on the stomach. Certain muscles may be relaxed more effectively while lying on the stomach or side, or while lying on all fours over a beach ball, rocking rhythmically forward and backward.

Standing Wedge for Ankle Dorsiflexion, Heel Cord Stretch

Materials

One 54 inch by 14 inch by 3/4 inch (137.2 cm × 34.8 cm × 1.9 cm) wood plank. (Plywood—good 2 sides). Two 12 inch (30.4 cm) piano hinges (with screws). Two 42 inch (106.7 cm) length 3/8 inch (1.0 cm) wood stripping. A saw, hammer and screwdriver. Two 18 inch × 14 inch sheets of adhesive-non-slip rubber material.

Construction

Divide the 54 inch (137.2 cm) plank into an 18 inch long standing surface, an 18 inch long base and a 7 inch long swinging support. Cut the ends of the swinging support at 45° parallel angles to permit easier movement. Cut six 14 inch long pieces of wood stripping.

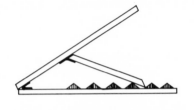

Join the standing surface end-to-end with the base by one of the hinges.

Join the flat side of the swinging support to the underside of the standing surface at 10 inches (25.4 cm) from the surface base joint. Nail the wood strips to the base so that their inner edges are at 8 inch (20.3 cm), 10 inch (25.4 cm), 12 1/8 inch (30.8 cm), 13 1/2 inch (34.3 cm), 14 5/8 inch (37.1 cm), and 15 9/16 inch (39.5 cm), measuring from the standing-surface base joint. This arrangement allows for adjustments of the wedge between 45° and 20° at 5-degree intervals. Reinforce each wood strip with two small screws. Stain the entire wedge and finish with polyurethane varnish. Glue and/or nail the non-slip rubber matting to the top standing surface at the bottom of the base.

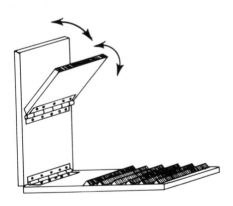

Figure 1. An ankle tilt board used for stretching the calf muscles.

Exercising in a pool may also be extremely beneficial because the buoyancy of the water allows movements to be performed with less energy expenditure and more efficient use of many muscles. We recommend using the pool for both stretching and **range of movement** exercises, which consist of easy, slow, rhythmic and flowing calisthenics that allow most of the joints of the body to move through their full stretching range. The pool temperature should be lukewarm, about 75 degrees; this may feel cool to some, but warmer temperatures are to be avoided as they produce fatigue.

Many MS persons have limited range of movement in at least some joints and muscles, and **the key to managing spasticity is to expand the number and kind of movements that can be performed**. The exercises should be done utilizing a minimum of effort.

Spasticity may also be reduced by the use of **relaxation techniques**, which involve a combination of progressive tensing and relaxation of individual muscles, accompanied by deep breathing techniques and imagery (see page 94).

In addition to the stretching exercises in the Appendix, it is suggested that the MS person read at least one of the exercise books published by the National Multiple Sclerosis Society. An individually tailored exercise program can be developed in consultation with a physical therapist. This can be carefully designed to meet individual needs and modified when and if one's physical status is altered.

Mechanical Aids

Specific devices can be made for individual patients to counteract spasticity and prevent what are termed "contractures", in which the range of movement possible for a given joint becomes restricted as the result of the spasticity. For example, a "toe spreader" or "finger spreader" are used to relax tightness in the feet and hands and to aid mobility. Braces for the wrist, foot and hand can be made to maintain a natural position and to prevent limitations on movement and deformities.

Medications

Lioresal (baclofen) is the most common anti-spasticity drug used in MS, and most patients respond well to it. The dose must be carefully determined for each individual; too little will be ineffective, and too much produces fatigue and a feeling of weakness because it interferes with the proper degree of stiffness needed for balance and erect posture. The correct dose is usually determined by starting at a low level and slowly increasing the amount until a maximum beneficial effect is obtained.

Lioresal acts by affecting the nerves that control the spastic muscles at their site of origin in the spinal cord. Another drug which is sometimes helpful in relieving spasticity is Dantrium (sodium dantrolene), which acts on the muscles directly. It is a very strong medication, and needs to be watched carefully. It can be helpful, but may induce weakness even at low dosages. Spasticity may also be reduced by Valium (diazepam), which is most often used for the relief of spasms that occur at night. Its calming effect also helps to induce sleep. Its strong sedative effect limits its use during the daytime. Valium must be prescribed with caution as it can become addictive if used too frequently. Another drug commonly used for spasms in the muscles of the back is Flexoril (cyclobenzaprine HCl). It acts quite specifically on these spasms, but may settle limb spasms as well. It usually works best when used in combination with one of the other spasticity medications. After taking any of these drugs for a prolonged period, they may become less effective (referred to as the development of "tolerance"), and it may be necessary to stop taking them for a period of time, after which they may again become effective.

MS persons very occasionally develop what are termed "paroxysmal" or "tonic" spasms, in which an entire arm or leg may draw up or out in a stiff, clenched or extended position. Tegretol (carbamepazine) is generally used to control such spasms, although Lioresal may also be quite effective. Cortisone may decrease spasticity in general, and is quite effective for paroxysmal spasms when used on a short term basis, but its long term use is not advocated because of numerous risks (see page 7).

Surgical Management

Occasionally, severe "flexor spasms" may develop, in which the legs are drawn up to the stomach in a painful spasm. If drugs are not effective in controlling these spasms, nerves controlling specific muscles of the leg may be destroyed with phenol, a chemical that is injected into the muscle or even into the spinal canal. This is called a "motor point block".

It produces flaccidity in the muscles, a profound looseness that is the opposite of spasticity. This relaxation may be more comfortable, but it does not increase functional mobility. A temporary loss of control over the bladder and bowel may be produced by phenol, but function usually returns in time. This approach is used only for the most severe spasms that do not respond to drug management. Other possible ways that severe spasms may be managed include surgical procedures that involve cutting nerves or tendons to decrease the contraction of specific muscles that are producing a major degree of stiffness.,

Generally, the faithful use of an exercise program and the appropriate use of drugs when needed will significantly increase the level of function, and avoid the development of these more severe problems.

CONTRACTURES

A contracture is a "freezing" of a joint so that it can no longer bend through its full range of motion. It occurs when the joint has not been kept mobile, usually as the result of spasticity. If a joint does develop a contracture, it becomes useless and often painful.

All of the approaches used to treat spasticity play a role in the management of contracture. The joint must be slowly mobilized, sometimes using heat or ice applied just prior to stretching to ease pain and allow more efficient stretching. Special equipment such as a tilt board is helpful. Lioresal (baclofen), Valium (diazepam), Dantrium (dantrolene) and Flexoril (cyclobenzoprine HCl) can be administered to decrease muscle tone and permit faster relief from the contracture. Occasionally, cortisone is injected directly into the joint to decrease inflammation and increase mobility. Braces may be designed to slowly stretch the joint; by changing the angle of the brace over time, a frozen joint may sometimes become mobile. In extreme conditions, surgery may be required to release the muscle tendons to allow the joint to move.

Joints usually freeze into the contracted position, but they occasionally become fixed in the extended or straight position. While this is usually less of a problem in terms of overall function, it is not considered an acceptable outcome, and this type of frozen joint is generally treated in a similarly aggressive manner as a contracted one.

Symptom Management in Multiple Sclerosis.
Randall T. Schapiro, M.D.;
© 1987 Demos Publications, New York.

TREMOR

Randali T. Schapiro, M.D.
Lisa Harris, O.T.R.
Mary Lenling, O.T.R.

The term "tremor" refers to an oscillating movement of the extremities or occasionally the head. As is true of all MS symptoms, tremor may come and go. It is one of the most frustrating symptoms to treat in MS. There are many different kinds of tremors; some have wide (gross) oscillations, while others are barely perceptible (fine); some occur at rest, while others occur only with purposeful movement; some are fast, while others are slow; some are of the limbs while others may involve the head, trunk or speech; some are disabling, while others are merely a nuisance; and some are treatable, while others are not. Because of this wide variation, as with all symptoms, proper diagnosis is essential before correct management decisions can be made.

THE MANAGEMENT OF TREMOR WITH DRUGS

The most common tremor seen in MS, and the most difficult to treat, occurs as the result of demyelination in the **cerebellum**. This is the area of the brain responsible for balance, sending its connections through the back of the brain (the brainstem) and the spinal cord. Demyelination in this area often results in a gross tremor which is relatively slow and which occurs with purposeful movement of the arm or leg.

This type of tremor is almost always exaggerated at times of stress and anxiety. The reason for this is not known, but this exaggeration by stress is true of most of the neurological symptoms of MS. One mode of managing the problem is therefore treatment with drugs that have a calming or sedative effect. For example, Atarax or Vistaril (hydroxyzine) is an antihistamine whose effect is to settle a minor tremor that has been magnified by stress. The anti-tremor effect must be balanced against the generally unwanted effects of the sedation by carefully monitoring the dosage until the desired effect is achieved.

Certain medications, such as phenothiazine tranquilizers, may cause a tremor to worsen, and on occasion they may produce a resting tremor that is gross and slow where none existed previously. While their sedative effect may be useful in the treatment of tremor, this different kind of tremor must be balanced against the positive therapeutic effects of the drug.

Because there is often a component of spasm involved in these gross tremors, the antispasticity agent Lioresal (baclofen) may provide some relief. The potential but reversible side effect of weakness must be balanced against the tremor reducing effect of the drug, again by careful adjustment of the dosage.

High doses of a drug used primarily for the treatment of tuberculosis, INH (isoniazide) can alleviate gross tremors which are influenced by posture. It is sometimes worth a trial if tremor is especially incapacitating, but high doses may be too toxic in a given individual to be used for this purpose.

Occasionally, a tremor seen in people who have MS is of a type called a **physiologic tremor**, also referred to as an "essential" or familial tremor. This is unrelated to the MS itself, and is very treatable with the drug Inderal (propranol).

OTHER TREATMENTS FOR THE MANAGEMENT OF TREMOR

Clearly, drugs are not the complete answer to the management of tremor. Physical techniques provide substantial relief in many cases, but results are mixed. Physical treatments fall into four general categories:

Patterning refers to a technique used by physical and occupational therapists to trace and repeat basic movement patterns. It is based on the theory that certain muscles can be trained to move in a coordinated fashion by repeatedly using the nervous circuit involved in a movement. These normal movements are guided and assisted by the therapist until they become automatic. Minor resistance is then added and removed, while the patient repeats the patterns over and over again independently. The muscles gradually appear to develop increased endurance for these learned movements, and manage to retain control when the patterns are applied to functional tasks.

Immobilization refers to the placement of a rigid brace across a joint, fixing it in one position and dampening the severity of a tremor by reducing random movement in the joint. Bracing is most helpful in the ankle and foot, providing a stable base for standing and walking. It may also be used for the arm and hand. The desired position of function is defined by the tasks that are to be facilitated, such as writing, eating, or knitting; the brace is used to immobilize the arm or hand for these tasks and then removed.

Weighting is the addition of weight to a part of the body to provide increased control over its movements. The general theory behind this approach is that more muscles will be used to stabilize a distant point in the body (hands, wrists, feet, ankles) when a heavier object is involved. This stabilizing action also tends to reduce the tremor and to provide greater sensory feedback to the brain. In practical terms, either the limb itself may be weighted, or the object being used may be made heavier, including utensils, pens or pencils, canes, walkers, etc.

Vestibular stimulation refers to increasing the amount of stimulation received by the "balance centers" in the brainstem, thus allowing the brain to function more normally. The techniques used challenge the patient's sense of balance by rocking, swinging or spinning, using such activities as sitting on a beach ball or swinging in a hammock.

These techniques are all used primarily for tremors affecting the limbs. Their goal is to teach the MS person to compensate for tremor by providing as much stability for the limbs as possible. It may be important to develop postural adjustments, such as using one's arms close to the body. Adaptive equipment and/or assistive devices that are nonskid, easy to grasp, and stable are helpful, and can be used for many activities, such as eating, writing, dressing, cooking, and homemaking.

Tremors of the head, neck, and upper torso are more difficult to manage than those of the limbs. Stabilizing the neck with a brace may be helpful.

Tremors of the lips, tongue or jaw may affect speech, either by interfering with breath control for phrasing and loudness or with the ability to voice and pronounce sounds. Speech therapy focuses on making changes that will increase the ability to communicate efficiently. It may involve making changes in the rate of speaking or in the phrasing of sentences. Suggestions may be made as to the placement of the lips, tongue, or jaw for the best possible sound production. In some cases, tremor may make it impossible to speak, in which case alternative communication devices must be used.

None of the techniques described above completely eliminates the problem of tremor. Their goal is continued function, which can often be managed by combining some of these therapies.

Symptom Management in Multiple Sclerosis.
Randall T. Schapiro, M.D.;
© 1987 Demos Publications, New York.

WEAKNESS

Randall T. Schapiro, M.D.
Andre DeLoya, R.P.T., M.S.

Muscle weakness due to loss of strength in a muscle or group of muscles can occur for many reasons and is seen in many diseases. For example, weakness in the muscle itself is seen in muscular dystrophy; in diabetic neuropathy the problem lies in the nerve that leads to the muscle; and in MS it is due to a problem in transmitting electrical impulses from within the central nervous system to the muscle. This transmission difficulty is the result of demyelination of the involved nerves, usually in the spinal cord, but occasionally within the brain.

It is vital that the source of the weakness be understood in order to properly manage it. For example, if weakness is due to a lazy, weak muscle, the muscle may be strengthened by lifting weights. However, when weakness is due to poor transmission of electrical impulses, lifting weights may only fatigue the nerve and further increase the muscle weakness. For MS people, it is important to realize therefore that **exercises that involve lifting weights or repetitive movements of**

21

muscles to the point of fatigue do not increase strength, they increase weakness. It is for this reason that exercycles, rowing machines, bar bells, etc., are not recommended without specific prior instruction.

It is impossible to separate the management of weakness from that of spasticity and fatigue. If muscles are less stiff, less energy needs to be expended in movement. Frequently, therefore, drugs or other treatments that lessen spasticity (see the preceding chapter) will also increase strength. Similarly, lessening fatigue may also increase strength.

Efficiency is the key to increasing strength with MS. Energy should be conserved and wisely used. This means using one's muscles for practical, enjoyable activities, and planning the use of time accordingly; for example, heavy activities should frequently be done before those that are easier to perform. The wise use of assitive devices may also be extremely helpful in increasing overall efficiency.

In some cases, muscles are weak simply because they have not been properly exercised, in which case exercise and overall activity are the best treatment. Repetitive exercises may also increase strength in the occasional individual who has a variety of MS that is not accompanied by fatigue.

Symptom Management in Multiple Sclerosis.
Randall T. Schapiro, M.D.;
© 1987 Demos Publications, New York.

FATIGUE

Randall T. Schapiro, M.D.
Lisa Harris, O.T.R.
Mary Lenling, O.T.R.
Jackie Metelak, O.T.R.

Fatigue is one of the most common and annoying problems for MS people. It is a difficult one to understand for others, since it is not manifested by a highly visible symptom. It can often be treated very effectively once its cause has been determined. Four specific types of fatigue are seen in MS, and sometimes more than one is found in a single individual:

☐ Fatigue #1 is the tired feeling that everyone has after working hard. It is a natural type of fatigue, and implies a good day's work rather than anything negative medically. Obviously, a good night's rest is the solution to managing this type of fatigue.

☐ Fatigue #2 is the "worn out" feeling that occurs when a person is depressed, often accompanied by poor appetite, sleep disturbances, and feelings of poor self worth. It is treated with antidepressent medications, frequently accompanied by counseling or therapy.

☐ Fatigue #3 can best be illustrated by visualizing a person with MS who walks three blocks, and has a slight limp after the first block, drags the leg after the second, and needs to stop after the third. Fatigue results because the nervous impulses that control the leg muscles are worked beyond their capacity. The best way to manage this type of fatigue is to allow for appropriate rest periods to allow a return of strength. It is as if one had a finite amount of energy to expend in a given time period, which must be managed and conserved to allow one to do all that one wishes to do.

☐ Fatigue #4 is a lassitude that is unique to MS, and the type that is meant by the term "MS fatigue". It is an overwhelming fatigue that can come at any time of day and without warning, so that suddenly one feels extremely sleepy and could in fact go right to sleep. The drug Symmetrel (amantidine) has been found to effectively manage this type of fatigue, although the manner in which it works is not yet understood. Stimulants such as Cylert (pemoline) and Ritalin (methylphenidate) may provide relief, but they have the unwanted side effect of causing difficulty in sleeping.

Occupational therapists are in many ways "efficiency experts", and their advice on planning, work simplification, and performing activities in the most efficient manner can help relieve all of the types of fatigue described above. Allowing for frequent rest periods is also helpful for rejuvenating the mind and body to enhance overall performance.

PRINCIPLES OF ENERGY CONSERVATION

☐ Balance activity with rest, and learn to allow for time to rest when planning a day's activities. **Rest means doing nothing at all**; there is a fine line between pushing to fatigue and stopping before it sets in. Rest improves overall endurance and leaves strength for activities that are enjoyable.

☐ Plan ahead—make a daily or weekly schedule of activities to be done, and spread heavy and light tasks throughout the day.

☐ Pace activity—rest before becoming exhausted. Taking time out for short five or ten minute rest periods during an activity may seem difficult at first, but it can significantly increase overall functional endurance.

☐ Learn "activity tolerance"—see if a given activity can be broken down into a series of smaller tasks, or if others can assist in its performance.

☐ Set priorities—focus on items that are priorities or that must be done, and learn to let go of guilt associated with not finishing tasks as the result of fatigue.

MINIMIZING FATIGUE BY CONSERVING ENERGY

The following are some specific suggestions for common tasks and groups of tasks that most of us need to do regularly. They take advantage of the principles described above, and are designed to conserve energy expenditures:

Kitchen and Cooking Arrangements

- Store items that are most often used on shelves or in areas where they are within easy reach, to prevent stretching and bending.
- Keep pots and pans near the stove, dishes and glasses near the sink or eating area.
- Permanently place heavy appliances such as toasters or blenders on countertops.
- Have various working levels in the kitchen area to accommodate various tasks, and evaluate working heights for maintaining good posture and preventing fatigue. Sit whenever possible while preparing meals or doing dishes, and use large stools with casters that roll to eliminate at least some walking. When standing for a prolonged period, keep one foot on a stepstool or an opened lower drawer, to ease tension in the back.
- Use wheeled utility carts or trays to transport numerous and/or heavy items.
- Use peg boards for hanging utensils to provide easier accessibility.
- Have vertical partitions placed within storage spaces to permit upright stacking of pots and pans, lids, and baking equipment.

- If storage cabinets are deep and hard to reach, use lazy susans or sliding drawers to bring supplies and utensils within easy reach.
- Use cookware designed for oven to table use to eliminate extra serving pieces.
- Use paper towels, plastic wrap and aluminum foil to minimize cleanup.

Meal Preparation

- Have good light and ventilation in the cooking area.
- Gather items needed to prepare a meal together, then sit while doing the actual preparation.
- Select foods requiring minimal preparation—dehydrated, frozen, canned, packaged mixes.
- Use a cutting board with nails to hold items that are being cut.
- Prepare double recipes, and freeze half for later use.
- Use electrical appliances rather than manual ones whenever possible, including food processors, electric mixers, blenders and can openers.
- Use a microwave oven or crockpot to cut down on cooking and cleanup time.
- Bake instead of frying whenever possible.
- Bake cookies in sheets of squares instead of using shaped cutters.
- Slide heavy items along the countertop rather than lifting them.
- Use a damp dish cloth, or a sticky substance such as Dycem to keep a pot or bowl in place while stirring.
- Line baking pans with foil to minimize cleanup, and soak pots and pans to eliminate scrubbing.

Cleaning

- Spread tasks out over a period of time; do one main job each day rather than an entire week's cleaning at one time.
- Alternate heavy cleaning tasks with light ones, and either get help or break major heavy duty cleaning tasks into several steps.
- Use a pail or basket to transport cleaning supplies from room to room to save on the number of back and forth trips.
- Use adaptive equipment to avoid bending, such as extended handles for dusters or brushes.

Laundry

- Wash one or two loads frequently, rather than doing multiple loads once a week.
- Collect clothes in one place, and transfer them to the laundry area on a wheeled cart if possible.
- If the laundry area is in a basement, plan to remain there until the laundry is done, and have a place to relax while waiting.
- If a clothesline is used, have it hung at shoulder height, and place the wash basket on a chair while hanging laundry.
- Hang clothes promptly after they are dry to minimize ironing.
- Sit down while ironing.
- Buy clothes that require minimal maintenance whenever possible.

Shopping for Groceries

- Plan menus before going to the store, and take a grocery list with you.
- Use the same grocery store on a regular basis, and learn where various items are located for easier shopping; a xeroxed master grocery list organized to match the store layout can be a simple way to minimize time and energy.
- Use home delivery whenever it is available.

Bedroom Maintenance

- Either put beds on rollers if they must be moved, or keep them away from walls.
- Make one side of a bed completely, then finish the other side, to cut down on the amount of walking involved.
- Organize closets for easy access, by making top shelves and clothing rods low enough to reach without straining.
- Use light weight storage boxes, hanging zippered clothes bags and plastic boxes for items needed daily.

Yardwork

- Alternate tasks and incorporate short rest period to avoid fatigue.
- Keep the garden small and easy to manage.

- Use adaptive equipment such as handles with extensions to minimize bending.

Infant and Child Care

- Always use leg and arm muscles rather than back muscles when lifting an infant or child.
- Wash, change and dress an infant at counter height.
- Kneel while washing a child in a bathtub.
- Use disposable diapers.
- Adapt the fasteners on a child's clothing for easier dressing.
- Have a child stand on a footstool while helping him/her dress or wash.

Sitting and Desk Work

- Arrange the desk and chair heights to facilitate maintaining proper posture, reducing slumping of the shoulders and neck flexion.
- Use a chair with good back support.
- Arrange your office so that your file cabinets, computer terminal, etc., are easily accessible.
- Use small lazy susans on the desk top for pens, paperclips, tape, stapler, etc.
- Use a phone device that allows the receiver to rest on the shoulder and frees the use of the hands during extended conversations.

Dressing

- Lay out clothing items for the next day before retiring.
- Sit while dressing whenever possible.
- When dressing, dress the weaker side first; when undressing, undress the strong side first.
- Use a long-handled shoe horn.

Bathing

- Organize shampoo, soaps, etc., and keep them together by the bathtub or shower.
- Use grab bars to assist in safely getting in and out of the bathtub.
- Use a tub bench or stool while showering or bathing.
- Always avoid hot water while bathing, since it increases fatigue.

Symptom Management in Multiple Sclerosis.
Randall T. Schapiro, M.D.;
© 1987 Demos Publications, New York.

WALKING (AMBULATION)

Movement impairment is a problem frequently associated with multiple sclerosis, and difficulties in walking represent one major type of such impairment. It is fitting that this section follows those dealing with weakness, spasticity, and tremor, because walking becomes difficult as the result of losses in strength, muscle tone, and balance.

When foot muscles are weak, a "foot drop" results, in which the toes of the weak foot touch the ground before the heel, producing a disruption in balance. As discussed in the section dealing with weakness, there is no way to strengthen a weakened foot, and compensation techniques become essential.

It is particularly important to wear proper shoes. A leather soled tie shoe is recommended. The tie gives maximum stability to the foot, and the smooth leather sole prevents the sticking that can occur with crepe or similar types of soles, which throws the walker off balance. It is understood that leather soles will wear over time and need to be replaced, but their advantages far outweigh this minor problem. A plastic (polypropylene) insert is often added to the shoe to keep the foot from dropping. This light weight brace (an ankle-foot orthosis, or AFO) picks up the foot and allows it to follow through in the normal heel-foot manner.

AFOs can also be designed to decrease spasticity, by tilting the foot to a specified angle, and to keep the foot from turning in or out (inverting or everting). Their proper use decreases fatigue while increasing stability. Such orthoses must be fitted by a specialist called an orthotist in order to provide optimal support.

A metal brace that fits outside the shoe may be needed if there is a significant increase in tone (stiffness) at the ankle. This is a "spring-loaded" device that keeps the toe from dropping. Fortunately, the development of new lightweight materials, including plastics and aluminum, has decreased the need to use more cumbersome and heavy metal (Klenzak) braces.

If the hip muscles as well as those of the foot are weak, the leg will be swung out in front to allow the foot to clear the ground. In order to maintain stability, the knee often is forced back further than it should be, a condition termed hyperextension. This movement puts significant stress on the knee. After a period of time, the knee will begin to hurt, and may become swollen as the result of arthritis. To prevent this condition from developing, a metal device called a Swedish Hyper-extension Cage can be fashioned to prevent the knee from snapping back. Alternatively, a custom made knee brace may be necessary.

With the aid of such devices, walking with less fatigue may again become realistic. However, if balance is also a problem, another assistive device such as a cane may be needed. Braces, canes and crutches are examples of "tools". They should be looked upon as tools in the same manner as a hammer or a drill is to a carpenter. It is wrong to feel that one is "giving in" to a cane or a brace. If a carpenter wishes to drill a hole, he uses the proper drill or the hole will be wrong. If a person with impaired mobility does not use the right tool, the job of walking cannot be accomplished. There should be nothing emotional about assistive devices—they are simply tools for improving mobility.

A cane is usually carried in the hand **opposite** the weak leg. The activity of walking is a "reciprocal" one, that is the left hand goes forward with the right foot and vice versa. When walking with a cane, it precedes or accompanies the weak leg. Walking with a cane on the weak side may cause a noticeable limp.

If weakness is pronounced in both legs, two canes may be needed. The same reciprocal pattern still applies, i.e., the left foot and right hand go forward together; the right foot and left hand go together. Walking in this fashion is slower, but there are always three points on the ground to provide increased balance and stability.

When walking stairs, the saying that applies is "up with the good, and down with the bad". Step up first with the strong leg when climbing stairs, and step down first with the weak leg when descending. This pattern makes the strong leg do all the work of lifting and lowering. Again, the cane should accompany or precede the weak leg. Always use a railing when possible. If it is on the same side as the cane, merely shift the cane to the other hand and use the stair walking pattern described.

If balance and weakness are more severe, it may be necessary to use forearm (Loftstrand) crutches. They provide greater stability than a standard cane, and do not require as much strength in the upper extremities. The walking patterns discussed for walking with a cane apply equally to walking with forearm crutches.

If balance is especially poor, a walker may be the proper assistive tool. The usual pattern to be used is: walker forward at arms' length, weak leg, then strong leg. Take normal steps and avoid stepping past the front of walker.

To measure the proper height for all assistive devices, place the device six inches away from the side of the foot and adjust the handles so that the elbow is bent approximately 25 degrees. As with any special tools, it is important to have the right ones, have them fit properly, and know how to use them correctly. An experienced physical therapist should be helpful in assuring proper fit.

If walking is still extremely difficult or impossible despite the selection of excellent devices, a wheelchair may be the correct choice. One should not fear the use of a wheelchair; it is in truth only another tool for mobility. There are many types of chairs, and selection is dependent on many factors, including the size of the individual, strength, and energy. Again, help from a physical therapist or a physician who understands the use of the chair is necessary to select the most appropriate one. When fatigue is a major factor, a motorized chair becomes the proper choice. There are many available, necessitating careful, educated shopping.

There is really no reason in today's world to not be mobile. The right assistive device coupled with the right attitude can make all the difference.

Symptom Management in Multiple Sclerosis.
Randall T. Schapiro, M.D.;
© 1987 Demos Publications, New York.

EXERCISE

Too often people with MS are told to rest and not overdo, and the fear of fatigue becomes almost unbearable. There is really no good basis for this fear. Proper exercise leads to increasing fitness and hopefully less fatigue. The process is slow. It all begins with a carefully developed exercise prescription. Like medicine, it should be prescribed by a professional who knows how to fit the exercises to the individual, usually a physical therapist or a physician.

The role of exercise in MS has become somewhat controversial, partly because the meaning of exercise is misunderstood. To many, exercise is defined as stressing one's body to the point of pain, an approach whose watchwords are "no pain, no gain". But in MS it has become quite clear that if one exercises to the point of "pain", fatigue sets in and weakness increases.

Rigorous exercise increases the core body temperature (as opposed to superficial skin temperature). In MS, because the nerves have had their protective shielding destroyed, this rise in temperature increases the short-circuiting in the central nervous system and further increasing weakness. Thus it is fairly obvious why exercise originally fell into bad repute with those knowledgeable about MS.

Our understanding of what is "good" exercise for people with MS, and how they should train, has increased considerably in the past few years, as the concept of "fitness" has developed. Fitness implies general, overall health. It is a wholistic concept that strives for improvement in function of the heart, lungs, muscles, and other organs. It is attained by having a proper diet, not smoking, and exercising appropriately.

Two major concepts underlie the term "appropriate" exercise. First, because of the wide variability of the disease, what is "good" exercise for one person may not be good exercise for another. **It is important to tailor an exercise program for each individual, rather than to have a set program for everyone who has the disease.** The second is that there are many kinds of exercise—all too often it is assumed that exercise refers only to running or jumping or similar types of activities.

Exercises that increase mobility through stretching and maintaining range of motion are discussed in the chapter on spasticity (see page 12), and a series of basic exercises are given in the Appendix. When muscles are stiff, more work is required to move them. This results in early fatigue and increased weakness. Thus these exercises play an important part in combatting weakness, by reducing the stiffness so commonly present with MS.

Balance exercises are discussed in the section on tremor (see page 19). These exercises are very different from those used to reduce spasticity. If balance is a problem, muscles must use more energy to maintain an upright stance. Anything that increases balance will therefore reduce weakness.

Relaxation exercises are discussed in the chapter Adapting to MS (see page 94). A person who is under stress will have increased weakness, and thus one cannot ignore techniques for learning how to relax in an overall program designed to reduce weakness and fatigue.

Aerobic exercises are the exercises most people associate with exercising. They may involve a bicycle, a rowing machine, a treadmill, brisk walking, running, or a brisk self wheel in a wheelchair. It is important to understand that the word "aerobic" implies that the body is taking in enough oxygen to meet its needs in the exercise program. This is compared to the "anaerobic" state that occurs when a person exercises too aggressively, starving the body for oxygen. **Endurance increases slowly but surely under aerobic conditions.**

Specifically, during any aerobic exercise, (except perhaps swimming) one should be able to speak a sentence out loud. Enough air should be available to permit clear and somewhat effortless speaking. If a person cannot speak in this fashion, it is highly likely that the type and/or extent of exercising is anaerobic and harmful.

The proper exercise prescription takes into account that each exercise should not bring on pain. **"No pain, no gain" is absolutely the wrong approach to exercise for the MS person.** The proper exercise prescription is a balanced one that includes many different types of exercises with the goal of improving the all around condition. With such an improvement, a gain of strength would be no surprise.

Symptom Management in Multiple Sclerosis.
Randall T. Schapiro, M.D.;
© 1987 Demos Publications, New York.

DIET AND NUTRITION

Esther Motyka, B.S., R.D.

Good nutrition is defined as the provision of protein, carbohydrates, fats, vitamins, minerals, water and cellulose (dietary fiber) in sufficient amounts to meet the metabolic needs of an individual. Nutrients 1) provide energy, 2) build and repair tissues, and 3) regulate and control the body's "metabolism", the sum of all body processes that sustain life.

NUTRIENTS NEEDED FOR GOOD NUTRITION

Carbohydrate is used primarily to meet the body's energy needs. Nutritious "complex" carbohydrates include breads, cereals, grains, dried peas and legumes, potatoes, and other vegetables, while "simple" carbohydrates include cakes, candies, pastries, sweets, etc. Carbohydrates, primarily the complex ones, should provide 50-60% of the calories in an individual's diet.

Protein has as its major function the maintenance, repair and growth of tissues. Both animal and vegetable sources provide proteins; those sources which contain all the essential amino acids, the "building blocks" of protein, are termed "complete" and those which may lack an essential amino acid, partially or totally, are termed "incomplete". Protein should provide approximately 20% of the total calories in the diet.

Fat is an important storage form of energy, and functions as the body's energy source after carbohydrate has been used up; when excess carbohydrate is consumed it is converted to and stored as fat. Fats contain "essential fatty acids" needed by the body for growth and healthy skin. Fat should not provide more than 20-30% of the total calories in the diet.

Water constitutes approximately 2/3 of the body's weight and is a major component of all cells and tissues. It also functions to 1) transport nutrients, 2) lubricate joints and the digestive tract, 3) assist in chemical reactions, and 4) aid in the regulation of body temperature. Approximately one liter of water should be drunk per 1000 calories consumed, at least 6-8 cups per day.

Minerals are inorganic elements needed in very small amounts, to perform vital roles in the body. At least 21 minerals have very specific functions in the body.

Vitamins are involved in a variety of metabolic processes in the body.

Cellulose or *dietary fiber* occurs naturally in foods of plant origin. It makes the stool bulky and soft, and decreases the time required for food and waste materials to pass through the intestinal tract. The topic of fiber is discussed in detail in the chapter on bowel (see page 61).

DIET THERAPIES FOR MULTIPLE SCLEROSIS

Numerous dietary regimes have been promoted for the purpose of treating or curing individuals with MS. **No evidence has emerged that any of them are effective.** some have been more well known, including:

The *MacDougal Diet* combined a low fat diet with a gluten free diet, encouraged a low sugar intake, and was supplemented with vitamins and minerals. With its many restrictions, it is hard to adhere to for very long.

The *low fat diet* was based on the belief that populations that consume a high fat diet have a greater incidence of MS. Animal fats were limited substantially, while various amounts of vegetable oils were allowed, especially those containing polyunsaturated fats. The diet also restricted certain canned, frozen or processed foods.

The *gluten free diet* was based on the premise that there was a higher incidence of MS in areas which produced and consumed wheat and rye, which are gluten containing grains. The diet omitted products containing wheat, rye, and some other carbohydrates, plus coffee and alcohol. Compliance with a gluten-free diet can be very difficult as so many food products contain wheat gluten.

The *allergen-free diet* was based on the theory that the lesions of MS may be some type of an allergic reaction to common allergens. It eliminated those foods commonly known to be associated with hives, skin eruptions, asthmatic attacks, hay fever, etc.

Regimens promoting vitamins, minerals, and other nutrients in amounts larger than normal found in the diet have also been offered:

As the term suggests, *megavitamin therapy* utilizes massive doses of vitamins. Its rationale is based on the premise that a deficiency in absorption or utilization of one or more vitamins is an underlying cause of MS. Megavitamin therapy can be expensive, and excessive doses of some vitamins, especially A and D, can have a toxic effect on the body.

Vitamin therapy, the use of individual vitamins or various combinations of vitamins, has been proposed based on the assumption of a possible vitamin deficiency in MS. Various vitamins alone and in combination with others have been tried, given orally or by injection with varying reports of success. Such use of vitamins is costly.

As with vitamins, the addition of various *minerals* to the diet has been suggested, including manganese, zinc and potassium. Many minerals may be toxic when ingested in large amounts over the trace amounts found in foods.

Polyunsaturated fatty acids (PUFA), including linolenic and linoleic acids, are essential fatty acids which are used by the body to synthesize other fatty acids and are also components of myelin in the central nervous system. Based on some studies which showed a low level of linoleic acid in the serum of MS patients, diets have been supplemented with linolenic acid, linoleic acid, sunflower seed oil, safflower seed oil, and even primrose oil. Some individuals may find the pure oils distasteful and prefer them in capsules, spreads or emulsions. Some people have been known to develop diarrhea when taking the supplements. The long term effects are unknown.

None of the above diets have been shown to prevent progression or exacerbations of MS, nor have an effect on the severity or duration of the exacerbations.

How does one identify a nutritionally inadequate diet or other false claim? Here are some basic guidelines.

☐ Does the promoter of a new claim propose a variety of foods in the diet, or does he rely largely on only a few foods and thereby eliminate important nutrient sources?

☐ Ethical scientists go thru their peers after experimentation for review, whereas questionable promoters will go directly to the public.

☐ Does the claim offer fast cures for diseases for which the medical community has none?

☐ Is there research to back up claims or is the information presented largely through "testimonials"?

☐ Does the promotor stand financial gain? Do proceeds go to an unknown "foundation" or other such body?

The promotion of self cures can be harmful when they prevent an individual from seeking competent medical help. When in doubt, check the facts with reliable sources of information, including:

☐ local colleges and university with nutrition or food science departments.

☐ local, state, or federal government agencies, such as the county extension service, state health department or the Food and Drug Administration.

☐ professional organizations such as the American Dietic Association (430 North Michigan Avenue, Chicago, Illinois 60611)

☐ local Dairy Council office or the National Dairy Council (6300 North River Road, Rosemont, Illinois 60018-4233)

☐ local hospitals, clinics, or public health departments which employ registered dietitians.

GOOD NUTRITION

The Basic Four Food Groups were developed as a simple device to aid in planning an adequate diet on a daily basis. The guide promotes a variety of foods, to assure an adequate intake of most nutrients. It provides the average individual with adequate amounts of all nutrients. The guide is a recommended minimum and may be adjusted upward as needed. Refined fats, oils and sugars are not included in the basic four groups, but considered an "other" category because they mainly provide calories and are usually not lacking in the American diet. The Basic Four Food Groups are described in Table 1.

Table 1. The Basic Four Food Groups

Food Group	Suggested Daily Serving	Major Nutrients Provided
Daily Group Milk and foods made from milk (e.g., cheese, ice cream, puddings, yogurt)	2 servings/adults 4 servings/teenagers 3 servings/children	calcium riboflavin protein
Meat group meat, fish, poultry, eggs, dried beans and peas, soy extenders, and nuts	2 servings	protein niacin iron thiamine
Fruit and Vegetable group dark greens, leafy or orange vegetables are recommended 3–4 times per week for vitamin A. Citrus fruit is recommended daily for vitamin C.	4 servings	vitamin A vitamin C
Grain Group whole grain, fortified and enriched products are encouraged, including bread, cereals, pasta and rice	4 servings thiamine	carbohydrates iron niacin

Symptom Management in Multiple Sclerosis.
Randall T. Schapiro, M.D.;
© 1987 Demos Publications, New York.

SEXUALITY

Kathy Harowski, Ph.D.
Lisa Harris, O.T.R.
Elizabeth Nager, M.S.W.
Randall T. Schapiro, M.D.

Sexuality is a complex part of life, one that is difficult to define or measure because its expression is special and private for each individual. It has its roots in being human, and adds a richness and pleasure to life that goes far beyond the sexual act, which is only a part of sexuality. While our society has recently become more open regarding sex and sexuality, many myths and negative attitudes still exist concerning the sexuality of those with chronic illnesses such as multiple sclerosis. Many people feel that a diagnosis of MS means that their sexual life has ended—that it is somehow wrong or "inappropriate" for them to continue having sexual needs or to seek information on maintaining a satisfying sexual life in the face of MS.

However, sexuality does and should continue to be an important part of life for MS persons. Sexuality affects one's basic feelings of self

43

esteem and views of oneself as masculine or feminine, provides pleasure and relaxation, and is an important part of relationships with spouses and significant others, since sharing a sexual life strengthens the attachment between partners.

A chronic illness such as MS can have a tremendous impact on sexuality. Sexual functioning—the actual physiology and mechanics of sex—may be affected by physical changes due to illness-related neurologic changes, or by the presence of symptoms such as spasticity, bowel and bladder problems, pain, and fatigue. The psychological feelings associated with coping with an illness such as MS, including anxiety and depression, may also interfere with sexual expression and desire. In addition, the partner of an individual coping with illness can experience a similar range of feelings, which may interfere with their sexual ability and interest.

While there may be changes in sexuality in reaction to MS, sexual needs neither disappear nor become inappropriate. This chapter discusses both the possible changes in sexuality and strategies for obtaining information and maintaining a positive sense of sexuality in the presence of the disease.

THE SEXUAL RESPONSE

The sexual response depends upon a complicated series of reflexes involving neuromuscular transmissions that are stimulated by a wide variety of visual, tactile (touch), olfactory (smell), and emotional sensations. Sexual excitement and response begin in the brain. Electrical signals are transmitted from the brain areas involved via the spinal cord to the sexual organs or genitals, through nerves that exit near the bottom of the spinal cord. The pathways between the brain and the genitals are long and complex, and there is a possibility that demyelination may cause a "short-circuiting" of them.

Impulses leave the central nervous system from the sacral spinal cord via the autonomic nervous system, which controls bodily functions that are considered "automatic" (see page 4). For example, this system controls the arousal that men and women experience without external stimulation, such as during sleep. In addition to these pathways, a center in the spinal cord mediates the arousal that occurs with more conscious thought, such as that involved in masturbation and sexplay with a partner.

The male penis is a tube of spongy tissue that contains a large number of blood vessels, encased by thicker, fibrous tissue. During an erection, blood flow out of the penis is prevented by a component of the parasympathetic nervous system (see page 4), thus increasing its length and diameter. The later stage of ejaculation, or emission of semen, is under the control of the sympathetic nervous system. With appropriate stimulation of the penis, ejaculation occurs as a **reflex**, meaning that it is under the local control of circuits between the sexual organs and spinal cord, with no or minimal control from higher brain centers.

Very similar processes occur in women. The clitoris is similar to the penis in its nervous system innervation. It and its surrounding tissues, the labia majora and minora (large and small lips), which comprise the external genitalia or vulva, have the same swelling response to stimulation as the penis during the excitement phase of sexual intercourse.

There are three well described phases of the sexual response in both men and women: 1) desire; 2) arousal, and 3) the orgasmic phase. During the desire phase, hormones are released that allow individuals to feel aroused and to respond sexually. During the excitement phase, a man's penis enlarges due to the blood flow changes described above, and a woman's vulva experiences a similar but less dramatic enlargement. As arousal proceeds to the plateau phase, maximal enlargement of both the penis and vulva occurs, with the woman's vagina providing secretions that lubricate the area. Following appropriate stimulation, orgasm occurs in both partners. Ejaculation is one of the main expressions of orgasm in the man, while in women it is expressed by intense contractions of the uterus (womb) as well as subjective feelings of pleasure.

SEXUAL PROBLEMS IN MULTIPLE SCLEROSIS

Given the complexity of the sexual response in terms of the neuro-muscular transmissions involved, it is no surprise that sexual difficulties are often encountered in MS. Frequently such difficulties are clearly physical, although a psychological component may be involved in many or most instances of difficulty.

Over 90% of all men with MS, and over 70% of all women, report some change in their sexual life since the onset of the disease. Men most often report impaired genital sensation, decreased sexual drive, inability or difficulty in achieving and maintaining an erection, as well as delayed ejaculation or decreased force of ejaculation. Women report impaired genital sensation, diminished orgasmic response, and loss of sexual interest; they may also be disturbed by intense itching, diminished vaginal lubrication, weak vaginal muscles, and a reflex pulling together of the legs (adductor spasms).

MANAGING SEXUAL DIFFICULTIES

The diagnosis of MS can alter one's image of oneself, and it is common to feel sexually unattractive and to be concerned about braces, wheelchairs, and catheters. Perhaps the single most helpful approach toward sexual difficulties is to focus on developing comfort with one's body, a goal that requires time and commitment. It is important to look for the positive qualities that one has as a person, and to put effort into feeling good about the self by taking care of oneself through exercise, diet, dress, etc. Feeling good about oneself helps defeat the myth that one has to have a "perfect body" to be sexy and sexually attractive.

Communication is critical to achieving a positive, enjoyable sexual relationship, and feelings must be dealt with openly and honestly. It is important to convey feelings about what feels pleasurable and what does not, and to experiment with different sexual positions and creative, alternative ways to give and receive sexual pleasure. Society emphasizes "normal" or "proper" ways to obtain sexual gratification, which tends to make sex goal oriented towards intercourse and orgasm. Many people find great physical and psychological satisfaction from those activities traditionally termed "foreplay". One excellent way to decrease or completely eliminate pressures and expectations is to become less goal oriented by renaming such activities as "sexplay". Sexual expression may be directed to parts of the body other than the genitals, increasing cuddling, caressing, massage or other forms of touch, and it may involve experimenting with oral sex, masturbation, vibrators, and other devices.

Emotional reactions may be an issue both for the MS person and his/her partner, as anxiety, guilt, anger, depression and denial are the natural consequences of coping with any chronic illness. Again, communication between partners is the key to managing such feelings. Couples should be sensitive to the fact that some painful feelings may not improve or disappear with communication and support. In that case, it might be useful to seek professional help in response to depression or anxiety that "will not go away".

To avoid bowel, bladder and catheter problems during intercourse, fluids should be reduced approximately two hours before sexual activity, and the bladder should be emptied before lovemaking. Be prepared in case an accident occurs despite these precautions, and remember that it is not a catastrophe. If a catheter is present, it can be taped over a man's penis or to a woman's abdomen. With or without a catheter, a vaginal lubricant such as K-Y jelly should be used.

Spasticity or leg spasms can be minimized by timing antispastic medication so that it is maximally effective during sexual activity. Having intercourse in a side position, with bent knees, or using pillows for support may make a difference and should be tried.

The use of a vibrator can compensate for a loss of deep pressure sense reflected as impaired sensation, numbness and tingling. A number of different types are available, including hand-held, penis shaped, and others.

If a man's erections are not sufficient for penetration or intercourse, surgically implanted prostheses may be an appropriate option. These include a rigid, noninflatable rod prosthesis and a semi-rigid inflatable device. Good results have also been obtained with the injection of papaverine, a drug that dilates blood vessels, directly into the penis just prior to intercourse.

While great strides have been made in diagnosing sexual difficulties and providing treatment alternatives, the key remains good communication between partners and between the person with MS and his/her health care team. By exploring options, requesting information, and seeking appropriate referral, a satisfying sexual life can be maintained while coping with the diagnosis of MS.

Symptom Management in Multiple Sclerosis.
Randall T. Schapiro, M.D.;
© 1987 Demos Publications, New York.

BLADDER

Cindy Phair, B.S.N., M.A.
Brenda Brelje, R.N.
Randall T. Schapiro, M.D.

Many people with multiple sclerosis experience difficulties in bladder control and urination at some point during the course of their disease. These symptoms can usually be controlled with medication to minimize any change in daily activities and lifestyle.

THE URINARY SYSTEM AND ITS CONTROL

Figure 1 is a diagram of the urinary tract, whose main function is to collect and eliminate body wastes in the form of urine. It is composed of:

☐ the **kidneys**, which filter the blood to remove waste products and produce urine at a rate of approximately one ounce (30 cc) per hour,

☐ the **bladder**, a muscular sac that stretches to store the urine until it is emptied by urination, a process technically referred to as "voiding".

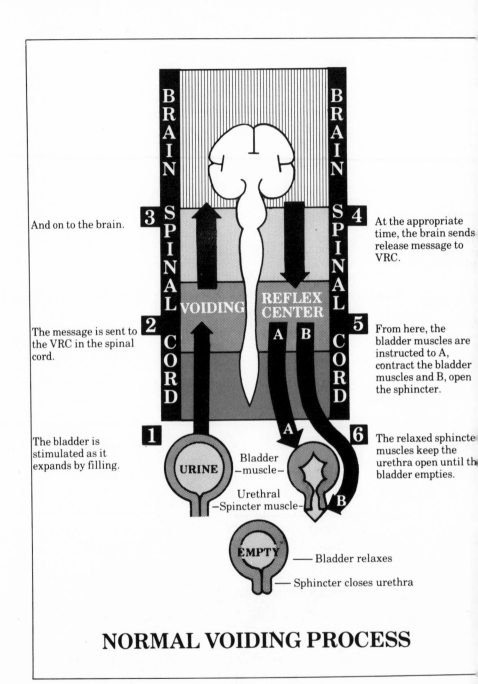

And on to the brain.

3 The message is sent to the VRC in the spinal cord.

2 The bladder is stimulated as it expands by filling.

1

At the appropriate time, the brain sends release message to VRC.

4 From here, the bladder muscles are instructed to A, contract the bladder muscles and B, open the sphincter.

5 The relaxed sphincter muscles keep the urethra open until the bladder empties.

6

B R A I N

S P I N A L C O R D

VOIDING REFLEX CENTER

A B

URINE

Bladder –muscle–

Urethral –Spincter muscle–

A

B

EMPTY —— Bladder relaxes

—— Sphincter closes urethra

NORMAL VOIDING PROCESS

Figure 1. (a) The urinary tract. (b) the small, spastic bladder. (c) the flaccid bladder. (d) the dyssynergic bladder.

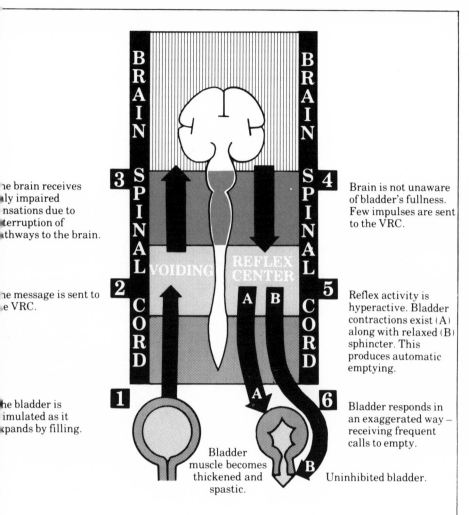

1e brain receives
1ly impaired
nsations due to
terruption of
1thways to the brain.

1e message is sent to
1e VRC.

1e bladder is
imulated as it
xpands by filling.

Brain is not unaware
of bladder's fullness.
Few impulses are sent
to the VRC.

Reflex activity is
hyperactive. Bladder
contractions exist (A)
along with relaxed (B)
sphincter. This
produces automatic
emptying.

Bladder responds in
an exaggerated way –
receiving frequent
calls to empty.

Uninhibited bladder.

Bladder
muscle becomes
thickened and
spastic.

VOIDING REFLEX CENTER

SPASTIC "SMALL" BLADDER

SYMPTOMS	TREATMENT
• URGENCY	PROBANTHINE
• FREQUENCY	CYSTOSPAZ
• INCONTINENCE	URISPAZ
	ORNADE
	DITROPAN

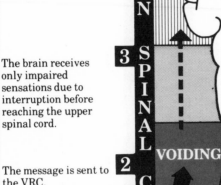

The brain receives only impaired sensations due to interruption before reaching the upper spinal cord.

3

Brain is not aware bladder's fullness. impulses are sent t the VRC.

4

The message is sent to the VRC.

2

VOIDING

REFLEX CENTER

5

Impulses are prevented from go to bladder—it is n under voluntary o reflex control.

The bladder is stimulated as it expands by filling.

1

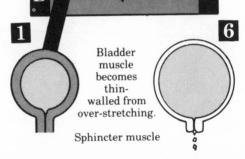

Bladder muscle becomes thin-walled from over-stretching.

Sphincter muscle

6

Bladder does not contract effective Over-filling can c dribbling.

FLACCID "BIG" BLADDER

SYMPTOMS

- URGENCY/HESITANCY
- FREQUENCY
- OCCASIONAL INCONTINENCE

TREATMENT

URECHOLINE (DUVOID)
VALSALVA
CREDE
SELF INTERMITTENT
   CATHETERIZATION

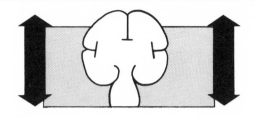

CONFLICTING OR DYSYNERGIC BLADDER
PROBLEM CAN BE ASSOCIATED WITH
EITHER *SPASTIC* OR *FLACCID* BLADDER
BLADDER MUSCLE AND SPHINCTER DO
NOT WORK TOGETHER NORMALLY –
RESULTING IN A COMBINATION OF SYMPTOMS:

EITHER

A BLADDER MUSCLE AND SPHINCTER
MUSCLE *CONTRACT* SIMULTANEOUSLY

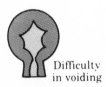
Difficulty
in voiding

OR

B BLADDER MUSCLE AND SPHINCTER
MUSCLE *RELAX* SIMULTANEOUSLY

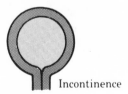
Incontinence

THE PRESCRIBED MEDICATION HELPS THE
BLADDER AND SPHINCTER MUSCLES TO WORK
TOGETHER PROPERLY

CONFLICTING BLADDER

SYMPTOMS: EITHER
- DIFFICULTY IN URINATING
  OR
  - INCONTINENCE

TREATMENT
- DIBENZYLINE
- BLOCKING AGENTS

☐ the **urethra**, a hollow tube through which urine passes out of the body when voiding occurs, and

☐ the **urethral sphincter**, a valvelike muscle that opens and closes to control whether urine remains in the bladder or is voided.

When 6-8 ounces (180-240 cc) of urine are present in the bladder, it becomes sufficiently stretched so that nerve endings in its wall are stimulated. These nerves send a signal of fullness to an area of the spinal cord called the "Voiding Reflex Center" (VRC, see Figure 1a), which in turn sends it on to the brain so that one becomes aware of the need to urinate. The brain sends a message back to the VRC that causes two signals to be transmitted, one to the bladder wall telling it to contract, the other to the urethral sphincter muscle telling it to relax and permit urine to flow out of the bladder.

BLADDER PROBLEMS ASSOCIATED WITH MULTIPLE SCLEROSIS

The elimination of urine by conscious choice is dependent on the integrity of these pathways between the VRC and the brain. A downward response by the brain to "empty" results in relaxation and opening of the sphincter, while one to "wait" signals the sphincter to remain closed. If the pathways between the VRC and the brain are damaged or interrupted in a disease such as MS, specific problems and/or symptoms may occur, the nature of which depend upon the location of the damage. If the connections between the VRC and the brain are completely blocked, the VRC will assume direct control of voiding and will stimulate the bladder to empty automatically. The most common bladder problems with MS are increased frequency of urination, urgency, dribbling, hesitancy, and incontinence.

Frequency involves an increase in the number of times urination occurs within the day; in some cases, voiding may occur as often as every 15-20 minutes, usually in small amounts each time. The frequency of urination depends on the rate at which urine is formed and the ability of the bladder to store it.

Urgency is the feeling of having to empty the bladder immediately, combined with an inability to "hold" urine once the urge to void is felt. People experiencing this problem have little time to get to the bathroom.

Dribbling refers to the leakage of small amounts of urine from the bladder. This may occur as the result of urgency and the inability to hold the urine. In some caes, the person may only be aware of this problem when damp undergarments are noted.

Hesitancy involves difficulty in beginning to urinate after the urge to void is felt. This symptom may be associated with urgency, so that one is unable to urinate while the urge to do so remains.

Incontinence is an inability to hold urine in the bladder, and may result either from not being able to reach the bathroom in time or from being unaware of the need to empty the bladder due to blockage of the pathways between the VRC and the brain due to scattered areas of demyelination. Despite the bladder's ability to stretch as it fills, it can only hold a maximum amount of urine and will empty spontaneously once this limit is reached.

Probably the most common type of bladder problem in MS results from a **small, spastic bladder**, sometimes referred to as a "failure to store" bladder, which results from demyelination of the pathways between the VRC and the brain (see Figure 1b). Due to the small bladder size, urine quickly fills it, stretching its wall and transmitting the need to void to the VRC and brain. Since the pathways to the brain are blocked, bladder emptying is no longer under voluntary control. Voiding then becomes a reflex activity, with messages to "empty" coming only from the VRC. A small, spastic bladder may produce symptoms of increased frequency, urgency, dribbling and/or incontinence.

When demyelination is located in the area of the VRC, a **flaccid**, or "big" bladder results (Figure 1c). The bladder fills with large amounts of urine, yet because the VRC cannot transmit messages to the brain it is unaware of this fullness. Since the VRC also cannot transmit messages to the bladder and sphincter, there is very little voluntary *or* reflex control over urination. The bladder fills and then overfills, producing symptoms of frequency, urgency, dribbling, hesitancy and incontinence. This situation is sometimes referred to as the "failure to empty" bladder.

The third type of bladder dysfunction is the **dyssynergic**, or "conflicting" bladder, in which the problem is related to coordination between bladder wall contraction and sphincter relaxation (Figure 1d), rather than the size of the bladder. In the dyssynergic bladder, either 1) the bladder wall contracts while the sphincter remains closed, resulting in a sense of urgency followed by hesitancy in beginning to void, or 2) the bladder wall relaxes while the sphincter remains open, resulting in dribbling of urine or incontinence. This lack of coordination between the bladder wall and sphincter is frequently seen in combination with either the spastic or flaccid bladder.

MANAGEMENT OF BLADDER PROBLEMS

Bladder problems can often be managed with medications and/or other approaches. In order to determine the most appropriate mode of treatment, it is first necessary to distinguish between the spastic (failure to store), flaccid (failure to empty) and dyssynergic bladder. This is easily done by carefully recording the frequency of urination and amounts of fluid urinated over a 48-hour period, followed by determining how much urine remains in the bladder after voiding. The amount of this residual urine is measured by inserting a catheter into the bladder after urination; a residual amount of less than 5 ounces (150 cc) indicates either a normal or small spastic bladder, while a larger amount indicates a flaccid bladder.

The small spastic bladder is best treated with medications that "slow" the bladder by decreasing the transmission from the VRC of impulses that cause it to empty. These medications include Ditropan, Probanthine, Cystospaz, Urispas, and Ornade. They lengthen the intervals between urination and decrease urgency, thus allowing more time to reach the bathroom and avoiding dribbling and incontinence.

Treatment of the big flaccid bladder is not as simple, and management frequently relies upon alternative techniques for bladder emptying rather than medication. One common method that facilitates more complete bladder emptying is **the Credé technique** of bladder massage. It involves applying pressure downward to the lower abdomen with both hands while bearing down, after as much urine is voided naturally as is possible; it is necessary for men to sit while using the technique.

If the bladder cannot be emptied sufficiently using the Credé technique, **intermittent self-catheterization** is used for more complete bladder emptying, in which a small tube, or catheter, is inserted through the urethra into the bladder to allow the urine to drain out. While initially this may seem to be a rather complicated technique, it is actually simple to learn and poses no risk. It allows a person to empty the bladder at planned intervals, thus avoiding dribbling or incontinence. The frequency of self-catheterization varies from person to person, but need not be done more frequently than every 4-6 hours. Medications such as Ditropan are frequently used in conjunction with self-catheterization to allow the bladder to fill more completely and decrease the need to urinate between catheterizations.

As mentioned above, conflict or dyssynergy is often combined with either a spastic or flaccid bladder. Initial treatment based on the 48 hour diary is aimed at either spasticity or flaccidity; if the techniques just described do not provide adequate control, it becomes apparent that the bladder wall and sphincter are not functioning in a coordinated fashion. Occasionally, formal testing with a "bladder analysis machine" is needed to accurately pinpoint the source of the problem. It may be helped by the addition to the treatment regimen of Dybenzyline, which improves coordination and increases bladder control.

If a bladder problem cannot be controlled with medication and/or intermittent self-catheterization, continuous (chronic) catheterization becomes necessary. This is done using a permanent **Foley catheter**, but this technique is only used when absolutely necessary because of an increased incidence of urinary tract infections.

URINARY TRACT (BLADDER) INFECTIONS

Urinary tract infections are an example of what is termed a "secondary" problem in MS, in that they do not directly result from the demyelination process; they occur as the result of, or secondary to, the retention of urine in the bladder. Mild infections may result only in an increased frequency and urgency of urination, while severe ones produce fever and generalized illness.

The incidence of urinary tract infections is higher than normal in individuals with a flaccid bladder, because bacteria can grow in the retained urine; in those who need to perform intermittent self-catheterization; and in those with an indwelling Foley catheter, which can provide bacteria a direct route to the bladder. Women are generally more at risk for the development of these infections than are men. The diagnosis of a urinary tract infection is made by a **urine culture**; urine is collected in a sterile fashion and tested for the presence of bacteria.

The symptoms of a urinary tract infection may include frequent urination, urgency, burning or discomfort when urinating, fever, or foul-smelling urine accompanied by the presence of blood or mucus. Since many of these symptoms are similar to symptoms frequently experienced by the individual with MS, treatment should not begin until an infection has been confirmed. Generally, an infection is suspected when symptoms occur suddenly or if fever is present. A urine specimen is cultured in the laboratory to confirm that bacteria are present before treatment is initiated with an antibiotic specific to the type of infection; the antibiotic is generally taken for 7-10 days.

Bladder infections can largely be prevented by complete bladder emptying, accomplished by self-catheterization techniques if necessary. Bacterial growth is prevented or retarded when the urine is acidic, which can be accomplished by taking high doses of Vitamin C. A person with a history of urinary tract infections can be helped by urinary suppressants and low doses of antibiotics. **Prevention is the key to avoiding bladder infections.**

☐ Urination should be frequent and complete, and holding urine in the bladder for long periods of time should be avoided.

☐ Women should be careful to wipe from front to back, especially after a bowel movement, and should avoid undergarments made of synthetic materials, which tend to trap moisture; women with recurrent infections should empty the bladder both before and after intercourse.

☐ Adequate amounts of fluid should be taken to keep the bladder "flushed", generally 6-8 glasses per day,

☐ Those who are prone to develop these infections should take 1000 mg of Vitamin C four times each day to make the urine more acid, since higher acidity inhibits bacterial growth.

☐ Those with indwelling Foley catheters should be especially careful to keep the catheter, tubing, and drainage bag as clean as possible, and the catheter should be changed at least once a month, using proper sterile technique.

Urinary tract infections can pose a serious threat to health if not properly treated, and it is very important to seek medical attention if symptoms occur.

When a urinary tract infection does occur, the key to its treatment is in the use of the right antibiotic, indicated by the results of the urine culture and a related test for the antibiotic sensitivity of the infecting organism. It is important that this medication be taken as directed **for the complete time period indicated** to ensure that all of the invading bacteria will be killed. It is a mistake to stop taking the antibiotic early because one feels better, because the remaining bacteria will reinvade and cause further problems.

SUMMARY

Bladder symptoms that may be associated with MS include increased frequency of urination, urgency, dribbling, hesitancy, and incontinence. These symptoms can be attributed to three different types of bladder problems. Their management is possible through accurate diagnosis and appropriate treatment.

Symptom Management in Multiple Sclerosis.
Randall T. Schapiro, M.D.;
© 1987 Demos Publications, New York.

BOWEL

Brenda Brelje, R.N.
Cindy Phair, B.S.N., M.A.
Randall T. Schapiro, M.D.

As is the case with the urinary tract, discussed in the last chapter, many people with MS have some degree of bowel complications at some point during the course of their disease. These difficulties can be effectively managed with medications and other treatments.

THE GASTROINTESTINAL TRACT AND ITS CONTROL

The gastrointestinal (GI) tract is a hollow, muscular tube that extends from mouth to anus and is responsible for the digestion and absorption of food followed by the elimination of the waste products of the digestion process.

The **stomach** primarily acts both as a storage chamber and the first site of major digestive processes. It slowly passes food to the **small intestines** and then on to the **large intestine** by a propulsive movement.

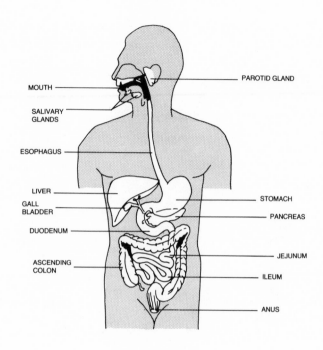

Figure 1. The gastrointestinal tract.

The large intestine is about five feet long, and is divided into four sections: the ascending, transverse, descending and sigmoid **colon**. In the sigmoid colon stool is concentrated into a solid mass by the absorption of much of the fluid that is present in other areas of the tract. The reflex process that leads to a bowel movement (defecation) occurs when stool moves from the sigmoid colon into the **rectum**, the last 4-6 inches of the tract (See Figure 1).

The rectum usually remains empty until just prior to and during defecation, when stool enters it either as a result of a mass propulsive movement or by voluntary contraction of the abdominal muscles. In a manner similar to what happens in the bladder to initiate urination, filling of the rectum with stool causes nerve endings in the rectal wall to transmit a message of fullness to an area of the spinal cord similar to the VRC involved in bowel function. As stool leaves the rectum, it passes through the **anal canal**, which contains the **internal** and **external sphincter** muscles. These sphincters, ring-shaped muscles that control the opening and closing of the passageway from the rectum, are normally contracted to prevent leakage. The internal sphincter is under the control of the spinal cord, and its relaxation is what is termed an "involuntary reflex" because it is not under conscious control, and its relaxation depends only upon stretching of the rectal wall by stool. In contrast, the external sphincter is under joint control of the spinal cord and the brain, so that if the time is not appropriate, a bowel movement can be consciously delayed by constricting the anus. In MS, the most frequently seen bowel problems are constipation, diarrhea, and incontinence.

CONSTIPATION

Constipation is defined as the infrequent or difficult elimination of stool. It is by far the most common bowel problem seen with MS, and may result in one or a combination of things directly or indirectly the result of the disease.

☐ Demyelination in the brain and/or spinal cord can interfere with the nerve transmission necessary for normal defecation, in a fashion similar to that described in the chapter on the urinary tract. A slower than normal passage of stool through the bowel results in more water removed from it than is normally the case, producing hard, constipating stool.

☐ A person with MS may limit his/her fluid intake because of a bladder difficulty. If fluid intake is not sufficient to allow the body to meet its basic needs, more water will be absorbed as the stool passes through the colon, also producing hard, compacted stool that is difficult to pass.

☐ Weakness, spasticity or fatigue may significantly limit physical activity, which in turn produces a slowing of bowel activity and movement of stool through the GI tract; again, more water will be absorbed from the stool, causing it to harden and become difficult to pass.

The Development of Good Bowel Habits

Dietary Management

Good eating habits are important to achieving good bowel control; a routine is important, and balanced meals should be taken at regular times in a relaxed atmosphere. The following should be eaten as a minimum each day: 2 servings of milk, 4 servings of breads and cereals, 4 servings of fruits and vegetables, and 2 servings of meat.

The intake of adequate amounts of liquid, 8-12 cups daily, and the addition of fiber to the diet will generally alleviate constipation. Dietary fiber is that portion of plant materials which is resistant to digestion; its addition to the diet aids in softer stool formation and decreases the amount of time required to pass through the intestinal tract.

A high fiber diet includes whole grain breads and cereals, raw fruits and vegetables, nuts and seeds, including cornmeal, cracked and whole wheat, barley, graham, wild and brown rice, bran (one of the most concentrated sources of dietary fiber).

To begin to increase the amount of fiber in the diet, it should include on a daily basis:

☐ one serving of fruit (with the skin left on) or vegetable, served cooked, raw or dried,

☐ one-half to one serving of whole wheat or rye bread, or fruit juice,

☐ one serving of bran (1 tablespoon), bran cereal, shredded wheat, nuts or seeds; raw bran may be eaten plain, mixed with cereal, applesauce, soups, yogurt, casseroles, or added to flour in cooking or baking.

If bran and other high fiber foods are incorporated into the diet too quickly, gas and distention, and occasionally diarrhea may occur. These effects can be eliminated or lessened substantially if high fiber foods are incorporated in small amounts and then gradually increased.

Establishing a Bowel Program

Because decreased sensation in the rectal area in MS can decrease perception of the need to have a bowel movement, stool may remain in the rectum and become hard and constipating. Although this and other factors can lead to constipation becoming a significant problem, it is manageable with a commitment to following an established routine of elimination, timing of meals, fluid intake and the use of medications.

The first step in establishing a bowel program is to select the time that is most convenient for having a bowel movement. While this varies depending on job commitments, family routines and other daily activities, the most effective time to have a bowel movement is shortly following a meal, since there is normally a greater movement of contents through the bowel at that time. With this in mind, 15-30 minutes of uninterrupted time should be scheduled in which to have a bowel movement.

Once a convenient time has been selected, it is important to adhere to this routine daily, whether or not there is an urge to defecate. Drinking a cup of warm liquid, such as coffee, tea or water, frequently facilitates the process. Although initially this schedule may produce little result, it is imperative that the routine be adhered to if a successful bowel program is to be established.

Medications

Medications may be needed if constipation cannot be corrected by changing the diet, increasing fluid intake and/or establishing a routine. To determine the most appropriate medication, the reason for the constipation must be determined, as it may be produced by lack of bulk, hard stools or difficulty in expelling stool.

If the cause of the constipation is inadequate bulk in the diet and stool, **bulk formers** can be prescribed. These add substance to the stool by increasing its bulk and water content. In order to be effective, bulk formers should be taken with one or two glasses of liquid; this combination distends the gastrointestinal tract, which in turn increases the passage of stool through the tract. Defecation usually occurs within 12-24 hours, although it may in some cases be delayed for up to 3 days. Daily use of bulk formers is necessary for maximum effectiveness; they are non habit-forming, so frequent use is not a problem. Common bulk formers include:

☐ Metamucil, taken in a dose of 1-2 tsp daily mixed in a glass of water or juice and followed with an extra glass of fluid. This may be increased to 1 tsp taken two or three times per day if necessary;

☐ Perdiem Plain, taken in a dose of 1-2 rounded tsp daily; it should be placed in the mouth (not chewed) and swallowed with at least 8 ounces of cool beverage, preferably more.

☐ Naturacil is a chewable, caramel-like bulk former; chew one or two pieces 1-3 times per day, following each with a full 8 ounch glass of liquid.

Stool Softeners

If the cause of constipation is hard stool, stool softeners are used to draw increased amounts of water from body tissues into the bowel, thereby decreasing the hardness and facilitating elimination. Consistent use is recommended to obtain maximum benefit; as with bulk formers, stool softeners are not habit-forming. They include:

☐ Colace (also known as DSS); take one pill every morning and evening;

☐ Surfak; take one pill every morning; and

☐ Chronulac syrup; take one ounce every evening, increasing to one ounce each morning and evening if necessary.

Laxatives (Oral Stimulants)

If difficulty in expelling stool is the cause of constipation, it can be corrected with laxatives, also referred to as oral stimulants. These provide a chemical irritant to the bowel, which increases its activity and thus aids in the passage of stool. While a number of laxatives are available over-the-counter, **care should be taken to avoid the use of harsh laxatives such as Ex-lax, Feenamint, Correctol, Dulcolax tablets, and caster oil, which can be highly habit-forming**. The same results can be obtained by using the following milder laxatives, which are less harmful to the bowel and induce bowel movements gently, usually overnight or within 8-12 hours:

☐ Doxidan; take one or two pills every night or every other night, to assist defecation after breakfast; these provide a stool softening action as well as a being a gentle bowel stimulant;

☐ Pericolace; take one or two capsules at bedtime; increase to two capsules twice a day if necessary;

☐ Modane; take one pill every night or every other night;

☐ Perdiem (not to be confused with the bulk former Perdiem Plain), which contains the bulk former found in Perdiem Plain plus providing a mild stimulant or laxative effect; take one or two tsp once a day, placed in the mouth and swallowed with at least 8 ounces of cool liquid, preferably more; and

☐ Milk of Magnesia; take one ounce at bedtime every other day.

Suppositories (Rectal Stimulants)
Rectal stimulants provide both chemical stimulation and localized mechanical stimulation combined with lubrication to promote stool elimination. These may be used either occasionally when necessary or on a routine daily or every-other-day basis, in conjunction with other medications already listed. Suppositories generally act within 15 minutes to an hour. They include:

☐ Glycerin suppositories, which contain no medication and provide local stimulation and lubrication for easier passage of stool. It is milder and less habit-forming than Dulcolax, and is used to help develop a bowel routine;

☐ Dulcolax suppositories, which contain a medication that is absorbed by the lining of the large bowel and stimulates a strong wave-like movement of the rectal muscles that facilitates elimination.

Enemas may be considered an occasional treatment for constipation, but **frequent use of enemas should be avoided**, as the bowel becomes dependent on them when used routinely.

In summary, many medications are available without a prescription for the treatment of constipation, but their indiscriminate use is to be avoided. A professional should be consulted to determine which medication or combination of medications is best suited to a specific problem. In attempting to control constipation, it may be necessary to begin a bowel program that includes a number of medications. this may seem rather overwhelming in the beginning, but as a routine is established and bowel movements become more regular, some medications may be eliminated. **Consistency is the key to regulating constipation.**

DIARRHEA AND INCONTINENCE

Diarrhea is much less common in people with MS than is constipation. It can, however, be a significant problem because there may not be adequate warning of an impending attack of diarrhea and incontinence may therefore occur. The probable cause of such diarrhea is a reflex-like activity due to the short-circuiting in MS that causes frequent emptying even though the bowel is not full.

The key to controlling diarrhea is to make the stool bulkier without producing constipation. Bulk formers such as Metamucil, Perdiem Plus or Naturacil may be helpful since they absorb water and therefore make the stool firmer. When used to treat diarrhea, the dose of bulk former should be no more than once a day, and one should not follow it with the recommended extra fluid as is the case when it is used to treat constipation. In extreme cases, medications that slow the movement of the bowel muscles, such as Kaopectate or Lomotil may be needed to control the diarrhea.

SUMMARY

Bowel symptoms that may be associated with MS include constipation, diarrhea, and incontinence. These symptoms are the result of both demyelination due to the MS process and to changes in lifestyle. Their management involves establishing a regular bowel program, and the use of medications as needed.

Symptom Management in Multiple Sclerosis.
Randall T. Schapiro, M.D.;
© 1987 Demos Publications, New York.

PAIN

While MS is generally a painless disease, about 20% of all MS individuals find pain to be a significant problem. It appears to result from what might be termed "short circuits" in the tracts that carry sensory impulses between the brain and spinal cord.

Trigeminal neuralgia, a severe, stabbing facial pain, is occasionally seen in individuals with MS. Treatment with Tegretol (carbamepazine) produces excellent results, apparently by calming some of the short circuiting in the sensory areas. To avoid its primary side effect of sleepiness, the drug is given initially at low doses and slowly increased to a point at which it adequately controls the pain. When taking this drug, the blood must be monitored at regular intervals to check for changes in the white blood cells. Other drugs that may be used to control trigeminal neuralgia include Dilantin (phenytoin), whose action is similar to but milder than Tegretol, and Lioresal (baclofen), used most commonly for spasticity. If drugs fail, a surgical procedure can usually be done that will eliminate the pain, leaving a much less disturbing numbness in its place.

The predominant type of pain seen in MS is a burning, tooth-achy type of pain that occurs most commonly in the extremities, although it may also occur on the trunk. The same medications used for trigeminal neuralgia are used for these burning "dysesthesias", but they appear to be less effective than they are for facial pain.

Occasionally, the use of electrical stimulation (TNS, transcutaneous nerve stimulation) over the area of pain may provide relief from pain. However, it frequently has the opposite effect and is therefore not often recommended.

Mood altering drugs (tranquilizers and antidepressants) may be effective in some cases, because they alter the interpretation of the message of pain. A number of such drugs are available, and with careful manipulation of the type and dosage some relief may be provided. In addition, biofeedback, meditation, acupuncture and other similar techniques may be of help in specific circumstances. Since pain is a symptom that clearly increases in severity when dwelt upon, a concerted effort to treat the reaction to pain is an important part of the overall treatment plan.

What is clear is that standard pain medications, including aspirin, codeine, and narcotic analgesics are not effective, because the source of pain is not the typical one that occurs with injury. **Pain medications are therefore to be avoided; they are not only ineffective but addictive.**

Low back pain is one of the most common symptoms treated by the neurologist, and it is therefore not unexpected that it is also relatively common in MS persons. MS itself rarely causes low back pain; it is more commonly caused by a pinched nerve or other problem. This situation occurs fairly frequently, because abnormal posture or an unusual walking pattern resulting from MS places stress on the discs of the spinal cord (padlike structures that cushion the areas between the vertebrae). This stress may cause "slippage" of the discs, compressing one or more of the nerves as they leave the spinal cord, and resulting in pain in the part of the body innervated by these nerves. Obviously, heavy lifting and inappropriate turning and bending will compound the problem. These movements irritate the spinal nerves, causing the muscles on the side of the spinal column (the paraspinal muscles) to go into spasm; it is this spasm that causes low back pain. If a spinal nerve is significantly irritated, the pain may extend down a leg to the muscles in the leg that are served (innervated) by that nerve.

If the problem is one of poor walking posture, the pattern needs to be corrected, and if spasticity is contributing to the problem it must be lessened. Local back care with heat, massage, and ultrasound waves are frequently helpful, and exercises designed to relieve back muscle spasm may be recommended. Drugs designed to relieve back spasms may be used, including Parafon forte, Flexoril and Robaxin, and some arthritis medications are frequently useful. If the problem is the result of a faulty disc, surgery may be needed to relieve the spinal irritation.

In the MS person, **spinal manipulation (rapid twisting or pushing of the spinal column) is not recommended** as it may irritate the spinal cord and increase neurologic problems.

It is critical that a proper diagnosis of the cause of any type of pain be made to ensure that it is properly treated. Diagnostic X-rays, including CT scanning, may be needed to pinpoint the cause of pain, after which the appropriate mode(s) of treatment can be prescribed.

Symptom Management in Multiple Sclerosis.
Randall T. Schapiro, M.D.;
© 1987 Demos Publications, New York.

SPEECH DIFFICULTIES

Speech patterns are controlled by many areas of the brain, especially the lower brain area called the brainstem. Depending upon the location of demyelinated areas, many different alterations of normal speech patterns are possible in MS.

If the cerebellum, the area of the brain involved with balance, is primarily involved in the existence of speech difficulties, speech generally becomes slow and fluency is diminished. Words may be slurred, but are usually understandable. If the tongue and throat muscles become involved, the speech pattern becomes still more slurred. In either case, speech therapy can increase both fluency and speech rhythm. While exercises are sometimes advocated, they are not usually successful for this type of speech problem.

Tremors of the lips, tongue or jaw may affect speech, either by interfering with breath control for phrasing and loudness or with the ability to voice and pronounce sounds. Speech therapy focuses on making changes that will increase the ability to communicate efficiently. It may involve making changes in the rate of speaking or in the phrasing of sentences. Suggestions may be made as to the

73

placement of the lips, tongue, or jaw for the best possible sound production. In some cases, tremor may make it impossible to speak, in which case alternative communication devices must be used.

Symptom Management in Multiple Sclerosis.
Randall T. Schapiro, M.D.;
© 1987 Demos Publications, New York.

VISION

The two major components of effective vision are the ability to image what one sees correctly, and the proper coordination and strength of the muscles that surround the eye and control its movements. Both may be affected in MS.

Inflammation and demyelination in the optic nerve, which connects the eye to the brain, produces **optic** or **retrobulbar neuritis** resulting in an acute overall loss of vision. It is often managed simply by waiting for the inflammation to abate, after which function will return. If the problem is sufficiently disabling, cortisone may be given to reduce the inflammation, either as a pill or in some cases by injection directly into the eye.

In some cases, vision remains imperfect even after the inflammation has been reduced. This is especially noticeable at night, when light is dim, although in normal light colors may appear "washed out". Leaving a light on at night may be helpful. Additionally, there may sometimes be "holes" in the vision, with part of the area one is looking at obscured. This cannot be treated with glasses, which only tend to magnify these areas. The problem can be adjusted to with time.

A weakening of the coordination and strength of the eye muscles produces double vision. It can be treated acutely with steroids, usually in a larger dose than that used to treat optic neuritis. With time, the brain usually learns to compensate for the double vision, so that images are perceived as normal despite the weakened muscles.

As is true with all symptoms of MS, great fluctuations can occur in visual symptoms. Visual acuity will often fall and double vision increase with fatigue, increases in temperature, stress, and infection.

Symptom Management in Multiple Sclerosis.
Randall T. Schapiro, M.D.;
© 1987 Demos Publications, New York.

DIZZINESS AND VERTIGO

The term "vertigo" refers to the sensation of spinning, which when severe can be accompanied by nausea and vomiting. There are many causes of vertigo. In MS, the problem usually results from irritation of brain stem structures that are involved in maintaining balance by coordinating the eyes, arms, and legs. The inner ears also play a major role in balance. Disturbance in the conduction of inputs to the brain from the inner ear may be very distressing. Dizziness and the sensation of lightheadedness are less severe than vertigo, but nonetheless uncomfortable. Obviously, other diseases which involve these structures will produce similar symptoms.

When vertigo or sensations of dizziness are relatively mild, antihistamines frequently provide relief, including Benadryl, Antivert, and Dramamine. Vitamin B (niacin) is occasionally used to dilate blood vessels in the hopes that this will make a difference. These medications, individually or occasionally in combination, will provide sufficient relief to allow the patient to continue functioning reasonably well.

Dizziness frequently accompanies an attack of flu. When flu and its accompanying fever and muscle aches occur, the flu symptoms are managed with aspirin or other medication; the dizziness often disappears as the flu symptoms ease.

If vertigo is severe, and vomiting prevents the use of oral medications, intravenous fluids are administered along with high doses of cortisone to decrease inflammation in the region that produces these symptoms, the brainstem area at the base of the brain.

Symptom Management in Multiple Sclerosis.
Randall T. Schapiro, M.D.;
© 1987 Demos Publications, New York.

PRESSURE SORES (DECUBITI)

Richard Werner, M.D.
Randall T. Schapiro, M.D.

Decubiti (literally, "without skin"), also called pressure sores or decubitus ulcers, are breaks in the skin that result from too much pressure on an area over a period of time. They are an occasional problem in persons with multiple sclerosis. They most commonly occur on the buttocks and other areas that are in constant contact with the surface of a bed or wheelchair. A person who has decreased skin sensation does not have discomfort to indicate that he/she has been in one position too long. Pressure sores frequently appear quietly, with little or no pain, and continue to enlarge, resulting in large holes in the skin that then expand into the underlying muscle. Additional factors that can contribute to this process include inadequate nutrition, dependency on certain medications, stool or urine incontinence, and lack of education regarding prevention.

When an area of skin over a bony prominence is continuously irritated, blood flow to the area is obstructed. When the pressure is

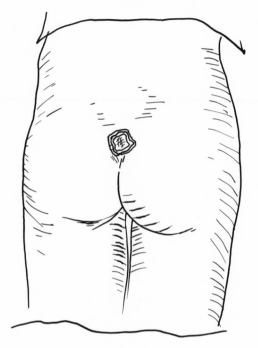

Figure 1.

relieved the body produces a "rebound response" of redness and heat. If the pressure is removed at this time the skin and muscle below can recover. This is called healing by first or primary intention. **Persons with MS should know how to avoid stressing the skin to the point that it cannot recover.** Several factors affect wound healing, including age, the presence of other medical problems, and nutritional state. The key to the management of decubiti is to avoid them!

Avoidance means transferring weight off contact areas at frequent intervals, without using pressure, shear, or friction to accomplish the move. It means using proper equipment such as foam pillows, air mattresses, water mattresses, and gels to disperse the weight of the body over larger surface areas. Foam rubber pads and sheepskins placed under pressure areas such as the sacrum (tail area) and heels will aid in dispersing pressure during transferring (moving). These "tools" plus proper positioning will relieve shear and friction. The skin must be frequently and carefully examined for areas of pressure and breakdown.

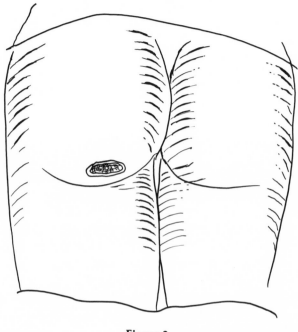

Figure 2.

For the bedridden person, the foam rubber or plastic sectional mattress may replace the standard bed. An alternating pressure mattress may also be used to relieve pressure. Turning once every two hours to avoid pressure to one area is important. The use of moisture absorbing sheepskins between the person and the mattress may also help.

If an ulcerated area should form, immediate attention is essential. No pressure should be applied to the area. The good skin near the wound may be toughened by applying Benzoin. It should be kept dry when the wound is irrigated with peroxide or saline. Many different "dressings" (bandages) are available. If the breakdown is minor, covering it with an "artificial" type of skin (polyurethane film dressing) such as Tagaderm may keep it from becoming infected and allow healing to proceed. Heat is often applied by an electric 100 watt lamp placed 18-24 inches from the wound for 10 minutes. After the wound is dry, it can be dusted with a drying agent such as cornstarch, aeroplast dressing, or even granulated sugar. If the breakdown is more extensive, the "Clinitron" bed protects all skin surfaces through an air-fluid system that eases pressure and keeps the skin dry.

The goal of treatment of a substantial ulcer is to obtain a clean wound prior to its closure. Surgery allows for healing by "secondary intention". Early surgical treatment is called debridement, which consists of trimming away the dead tissue. Unless the person has an infection, antibiotics are not routinely used. After and between debridements, frequent changes of the dressings, using wet-to-dry fluff gauze soaked in saline, are excellent for removing dead tissue from the ulcer. During this time the person's medical and nutritional status must be improved to facilitate healing and prevent a recurrence.

If more extensive surgery is necessary, several principles are followed: 1) the ulcer cavity (opening) with its surrounding scar tissue must be completely removed; 2) the bony edge must also be removed; and 3) the wound must be covered with good skin. If an ulcer is allowed to expand to a large area there is a risk of death.

Proper management of the person after surgery is critical for a favorable outcome. Care not to irritate the wound until it is healed is obvious. Following healing further attention to prevention is even more important.

If careful attention is paid the preventive measures described above, the chances of a pressure sore forming will be minimized. Prevention is the best strategy!

Symptom Management in Multiple Sclerosis.
Randall T. Schapiro, M.D.;
© 1987 Demos Publications, New York.

WEIGHT GAIN

Weight gain can be a problem in MS if a person's activity level drops but caloric intake remains constant. There is no data indicating that weight gain causes weakness, but it is not good for one's overall health and is unattractive. It can make general movement and especially aided transfers more difficult than need be the case.

Unfortunately, those confined to a wheelchair show weight gains first in the stomach. While stomach firming exercises may be of some benefit, it is not usually possible to do enough repetitions to cause an effective redistribution of weight, and a full stomach is practically unavoidable.

The same basic dietary guidelines that apply to everyone apply to MS people. A balance between exercise, calories and fatigue must be achieved. This starts with eating smaller meals. Many people find that eating small but frequent meals results both in lower overall caloric intake and greater satisfaction.

Symptom Management in Multiple Sclerosis.
Randall T. Schapiro, M.D.;
© 1987 Demos Publications, New York.

NUMBNESS

Numbness is one of the most common complaints in MS, usually appearing as an annoyance rather than as a truly disabling symptom. It occurs because the nerves that transmit sensation from the area affected do not conduct information properly, so that one is unable to feel sensations from that area.

There is little that can be done to treat numbness, and since it is usually a harmless symptom there is no real need to do so. Steroids may in many cases improve sensation through their decrease of inflammation, but their use is reserved for instances of real need.

Focussing on numbness can magnify the problem and make it especially bothersome. The best treatment for it is the realization that it is an annoyance only and does not imply a worsening of the disease.

Symptom Management in Multiple Sclerosis.
Randall T. Schapiro, M.D.;
© 1987 Demos Publications, New York.

COLD FEET

Cold feet is a common complaint in MS, often even in the milder forms of the disease. The maintenance of skin temperature is an "involuntary" process, one that is under the control of that portion of the nervous system referred to as "autonomic", which controls functions such as heart rate, sweating, and pupil dilation. Short circuiting in the interconnections that control the diameter of blood vessel and those nerves that sense temperature is responsible for the perception of cold feet.

This symptom can be annoying, but it is innocuous; there is nothing wrong with the circulatory system itself in the legs or feet, and there is nothing dangerous in the slight drop in temperature that produces this sensation.

Warm socks, electric blankets and similar local treatments are the best way to manage the problem. Occasionally, medications that dilate blood vessels, or the vitamin niacin, may be used to alleviate the symptom in cases where it is particularly annoying.

Symptom Management in Multiple Sclerosis.
Randall T. Schapiro, M.D.;
© 1987 Demos Publications, New York.

SWOLLEN ANKLES

Swollen ankles are the result of an accumulation of "lymphatic fluid", which helps to carry nutrients and other substances to the organs of the body. This accumulation most often results from reduced activity of the muscles of the leg, which help to keep the fluid in the "lymphatic channels" and propel it upwards. When the fluid leaks out of its channels, gravity causes it to pool in the ankles and feet. This is a problem common to many diseases in which the use of the legs is reduced. Unless the swelling is extreme, it is normally painless.

"Water pills" (diuretics) usually fail to reduce this type of swelling. Treatment is simple, and consists of keeping the feet sufficiently elevated that gravity can begin to move the fluid toward the trunk. This means placing the feet higher than the hips for periods of time during the day and all night. Support stockings may be of assistance by helping to keep the lymphatic fluid within its normal channels; these must be fit properly to avoid pinching the muscles of the leg.

Despite a continued leakage of fluid, swollen ankles are a nuisance requiring looser shoes, etc., not a sign of a major problem. The problem may be noticed more in summer, because blood vessels and lymph channels dilate (swell) to a greater extent when the temperature is higher.

Occasionally, extra fluid may accumulate in the body and pool in the ankles because the heart is not functioning properly. If a cardiac problem is involved, the swelling may be accompanied by shortness of breath, coughing, and a general feeling of being unwell. It is therefore important that a physician assess the cause of ankle swelling and determine proper treatment.

Symptom Management in Multiple Sclerosis.
Randall T. Schapiro, M.D.;
© 1987 Demos Publications, New York.

ADAPTING TO MULTIPLE SCLEROSIS

Randall T. Schapiro, M.D.
Mary Hooley, M.S.
Elizabeth Nager, M.S.W.

Adapting to MS begins when the first symptom appears. Usually it is vague—mild numbness, some tingling, possibly a feeling of weakness, occasionally some urgency of urination. The initial thought is to deny the problem and to ignore it. However, if the symptom persists, fear overcomes denial, often accompanied by self-directed anger. The fear is that of "going crazy", of believing that nothing is really wrong but it is "all in my head".

Often the opinions of several physicians are sought, including family doctors, internists, and neurologists. Some M.D.'s are vague about the problem, refraining from giving it a name, while some may mention MS. Stress and fear build until the tests are completed and the diagnosis is confirmed. Often this is followed by a sense of relief that the problem is medical and not psychological.

However, this relief disappears, and anger accompanied by grief once again surfaces. These feelings are often directed somewhat randomly, sometimes turned toward family, friends, or physicians as if they were responsible for the disease. A lack of understanding leads to more anger, fear, and resentment, and a "why me" feeling develops.

Some parallels can be drawn between the MS adjustment process and the stages of grief that people go through in dealing with the processes of death and dying, as described by Elizabeth Kubler-Ross in her volume *On Death and Dying*. She observed that people initially deny that death will occur. This is followed by anger, then by a bargaining stage, which in turn evolves into depression and then finally acceptance. The order may vary but the process is fairly constant. Family and close friends must also go through this adjustment process, and children in their own way may follow suit.

In the newly diagnosed MS person, as grieving evolves into depression, it is accompanied by loss of sleep, change of appetite and feelings of despondency. This sequence results from decreased self-esteem, changes in self image, life plans, goals, and values, and frequently a fear of rejection by family and friends. Resolution of these feelings is hoped for at the end of the cycle, accompanied by the feeling of peace that comes with the understanding that life must go on.

Dr. David Welch (personal communication) has observed the following stages of development in understanding MS:

1) Admission: the individual allows him/herself to admit the reality of MS. This admission is private, and involves no one else. Implicit in this admission is that from that moment on all relationships will in some way be altered.

2) Acknowledgement: eventually the fact that one has MS is reluctantly disclosed. Other people need to know if they are to respond properly to the person with MS.

3) Accommodation: the disease requires the subordination of some things to the requirements of others.

4) Adaptation: the environment needs to be modified to suit the conditions. The world needs to be changed to suit the person with MS, not the reverse.

There are a number of ways to deal with all the adjustments required by MS. The element of stress is constant throughout all phases of the adjustment process. Its effect on the actual demyelinating process is unclear, but in all likelihood stress does not increase demyelination. A flair-up of symptoms in a person under stress is not a true exacerbation caused by increasing demyelination, despite the fact that stress clearly enhances the symptoms caused by demyelination. While the brain has remarkable powers to compensate for the effects of disease, it often loses this ability when under stress. Symptoms that were previously compensated for will then be uncovered. The MS person will therefore appear to have increased symptoms and problems, which can in turn lead to more stress. It is therefore important that ways of coping with stress be developed.

Under normal conditions, stress usually forces one to change and readjust one's outlook. However, the chronic stress which accompanies a disease such as MS may instead result in continued decompensation and maladaptation. This only perpetuates the stress, and the stress-illness relationship becomes quite complicated. Simply put, the stress "feeds" the illness, and the illness "feeds" the stress.

All of this results in an angry and despondant person. Anger is what shows on the outside but depression is the internal mood. The person feels betrayed by his own body. The anger alienates others just when support is most needed. This cycle has lead to the perception of an "MS personality". There is no evidence to suggest that a specific personality exists in people with MS. Rather a loss of self esteem brought on by the perceived loss of physical function leads to mourning these losses, which in turn results in the development of personality traits that may be perceived as very different from that of the "predisease" state.

Very occasionally, the bulk of the demyelination occurs within the brain, and intellect ("smartness") actually decreases. Memory, planning, and foresight, diminish, and the personality changes. Initially these changes are subtle, but they increase with time. Emotional lability is the hallmark of this type of disease, with inappropriate episodes of crying and/or laughing. Older memories are lost last in MS, while remembering recent events presents the most difficulty. These changes are the result of demyelination rather than psychological causes. Thus counselling for this problem must be focused on understanding and adjustment. Counselling the family and friends can lead to better understanding. Antidepressants may help in controlling some of the emotional lability while tranquilizers are sometimes necessary to control behavior. **It is important to emphasize that while this type of MS exists it is very rare.**

Most life style stresses caused by MS will be helped by appropriate counselling. Many MS persons do not want to recognize the psychological component, and the counselling must be subtly offered or it will be strongly refused. Coping skills need to be developed on an individual basis. They cannot be easily learned from simply reading a book. They involve learning to deal effectively with stereotypes of the disabled in the community, perceived changes in masculinity/femininity, changes in relationships, changes of roles within the family, changes in employment status, increased dependence on others, and changes in physical condition.

Some practical coping techniques include:
- Making a list of conditions required for positive self-esteem, and disciplining yourself to create at least some of them.
- Determining a way (small or large) to contribute to society and follow through.
- Attending appropriate counselling sessions.
- Learning to say no to certain requests in such a way as not to damage self-esteem.
- Making a list of people who can be relied on for various kinds of support, and call on them for assistance when feelings of despair appear.
- Discipline, to stay as healthy and physically fit as possible.
- Creating opportunities for getting out of the house.
- Taking charge of situations rather than allowing them to dictate to you.
- Prioritizing projects.

RELAXATION TECHNIQUES

While stress is usually viewed as something to be avoided, realistically the key is to learn proper ways of managing that stress which is unavoidable. Some stress is desirable; it is energizing, helps to motivate us, and captivates our interests. The stress that must be managed is the "distress", which can hamper our ability to cope with the events and people in our lives.

Body and mind are linked, and stress affects both our physical and emotional well-being. Stress can produce physical signs such as knotting of the stomach, increased spasticity, headaches, tight or sore muscles in the neck, and an increased pulse rate. If left unchecked, more severe symptoms appear, such as insomnia, fatigue, anxiety, poor concentration, and poor problem-solving abilities.

Learning relaxation techniques provides a tool with which stress can be controlled, putting you in better overall control of your life and wellness. Relaxation takes practice. To be successful, one must learn to keep a passive attitude and to let go of thoughts that drift in and out of your mind. The following steps should be practiced until they become second nature.

- Begin by finding a quiet place where you will be undisturbed for half an hour or so.
- Sit with your arms, head, and feet supported, or lie down.
- Close your eyes. You may wish to turn on some soft music.
- Focus on your breathing. The goal is deep, steady, smooth and rhythmic breathing.
- Relax your muscles, by working systematically through your body. Tell yourself to relax your feet, calf muscles, thighs, buttocks, abdomen, chest, arms, hands, neck, and head. With each breath let your body become heavier and heavier.
- Now imagine yourself in a pleasant scene. Guide yourself to a fantasy trip where you always wanted to go or to return to. Explore this place with all of your senses.
- When you have spent enough time there, leave knowing that you can return at will. Slowly open your eyes and enjoy the calm.

Individual counselling is helpful when there is difficulty making the necessary adaptations, when there is a lot of anger, when depression becomes an ongoing problem, when self esteem fails, or when there is difficulty in accepting the existence of MS.

Group counselling is helpful when one feels that no one understands the problems, or when the support system is inadequate.

The person with MS need not go through life waiting for the other shoe to drop. By understanding some of the psychological changes that accompany chronic disease, an active role can be taken to achieve a healthy mental state. The physically challenged must also win the "mental/emotional" challenge. There is no simple way to do this, but what is clear is that if one surrenders, one loses!

Symptom Management in Multiple Sclerosis.
Randall T. Schapiro, M.D.;
© 1987 Demos Publications, New York.

GLOSSARY

ACTH—Adrenocorticotropic hormone, a hormone produced by the pituitary gland which stimulates the adrenal glands to produce cortisone.

Ataxia—The inability to properly coordinate movement. This usually refers to walking and to movement of the arms.

Autonomic Nervous System—That portion of the peripheral nervous system which is not under voluntary control. It governs "automatic" functions such as sweating, heart rate, sexual functions, and bowel motility.

Catheter, Urinary—A tube inserted into the bladder for drainage of urine.

Central Nervous System—The CNS consists of the brain and spinal cord. It is where many of the bodily functions (such as muscle control, eyesight, breathing, memory, etc.) are generated, processed, and signaled to the different parts of the body.

Cerebral Spinal Fluid—A water-like fluid which surrounds the brain and spinal cord.

Contracture—A decrease in the range of motion in a muscle due to stiffness around a joint.

Cortisone/Corticosteroids—Hormones of the adrenal glands known to have anti-inflammatory and immune system suppressing properties.

Decubitus—A break in the skin resulting from pressure on an area of skin for a prolonged period; a pressure sore.

Demyelination—The abnormal process of myelin destruction.

Dexamethasone (Decadron)—A high potency cortisone which is used to decrease swelling in the nervous system.

Diplopia—Double vision.

Dysarthria—Slurring of speech.

Exacerbation—A sudden worsening of symptoms.

Flaccidity—Looseness and accompanying weakness in an affected muscle.

Immune Defect—The general term describing different malfunctions of the immune system, in which it either does not respond to a foreign substance by destroying or neutralizing it, or where the immune system erroneously destroys normal structures of the body. Multiple sclerosis may result from such a defect.

Immune System—Consists of a number of different organs in the human body (lymph nodes, bone marrow, thymus, etc.) which produce certain types of white blood cells and antibodies which have the ability to destroy or neutralize various germs, substances and poisons.

Incontinence—The inability to control the urinary bladder or bowels.

Lesion—A structural abnormality in the nervous system.

Lumbar Puncture—A spinal tap, involving the insertion of a needle into the spinal canal in order to obtain spinal fluid, and/or inject substances into the spinal canal.

Motor—Usually referring to the ability to carry out activities which require the use of bodily muscles.

Myelin—A substance consisting of fat and protein, which acts as an insulator around most of the nerve fibers in the human body. It is found in the central and peripheral nervous system.

Multiple Sclerosis—A disorder of the CNS usually characterized by worsenings (exacerbations) and improvements (remissions) of symptoms. Multiple scars gradually form in the CNS. Most frequently encountered symptoms are loss of strength; difficulties with balance and bladder control; numbness and tingling; and blurred and double vision.

Neurogenic Bladder—A condition in which urinary bladder control is disturbed, which may manifest itself by frequent urgencies for urination, a loss of sensation for urge, an inability to empty the bladder even though the urge may be present, or a complete loss of control of the urinary bladder which then empties itself irregularly.

Optic Neuritis—An inflammation of the nerve which connects the eye with the brain, and which manifests itself mainly as blurring or loss of vision and occasionally pain.

Paresthesias—Sensations of tingling or "pins and needles" in different portions of the body.

Peripheral Nervous System—Consists of numerous nerves in the body which serve the function of carrying the stimuli and information into the brain and spinal cord and, from there, back into the different parts of the body.

Plaque—A scarring in the nervous system due to the destruction of myelin.

Position Sense—The ability to feel slight movements of fingers or toes.

Reflex—An immediate response of a certain part of the human body to a brief stimulus, which usually does not require processing of the stimulus through the conscious mind. An example is the jerking of the leg upon striking the knee.

Spasticity—The loss of normal elasticity of leg and/or arm muscles resulting from a disease process in the CNS. It is often manifested by extreme stiffness of the muscles, which results in difficulties with active and passive movements of the extremities.

Tremor—Various involuntary movements involving arms, legs or head, occurring in numerous illnesses and conditions and greatly varying in type and severity.

Urinary Tract—The pathway of urination to the outside. It includes the kidney, ureter, bladder, and urethra.

Vertigo—Dizziness, or a spinning sensation.

Symptom Management in Multiple Sclerosis.
Randall T. Schapiro, M.D.;
© 1987 Demos Publications, New York.

APPENDIX:
EXERCISES FOR SPASTICITY

Range of Motion—Lower Extremity

CAUTION—When doing passive exercises, do exercises slowly and apply pressure steadily, especially if extreme tightness is present.

1. Ankle Dorsi flexion (calf stretch) (Bending ankle up). Back lying

Grab the heel, placing the ball of the foot against your forearm, and bend the ankle up. (Push the toes toward the knee.)

2. Hamstring stretch (Hip flexion
   with straight knee). Back lying

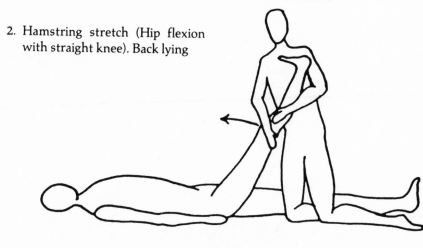

3. Hip flexion (knee to chest)
   Buttock stretch. Back lying

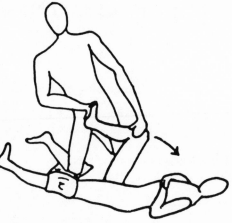

4. Internal—external rotation
   (rolling leg in and out). Back lying

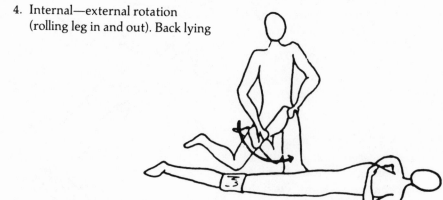

5. Abduction—adduction (out to side). Back lying

6. Knee flexing (front, thigh stretch) Face lying

7. Hip extension (leg backward at hip). Face lying

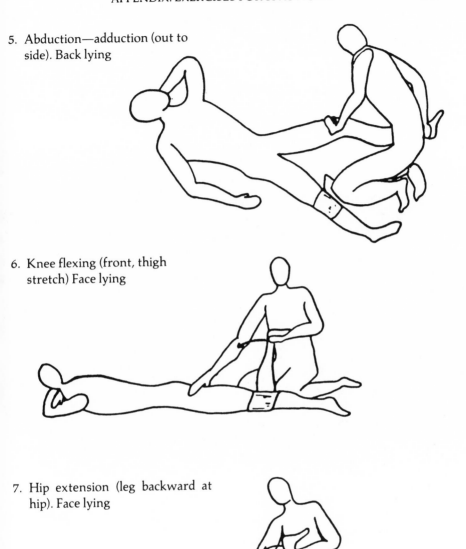

8. Trunk flexion—(back stretch)
   Bring both knees up to chest.
   Back lying

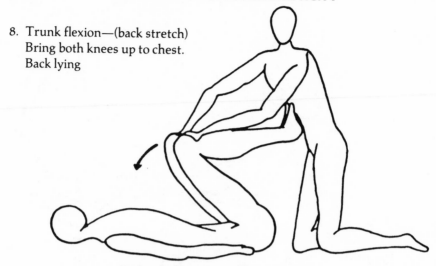

Independent Stretching Program

1. Heel Cord Stretch—Sit on a mat, the floor or the bed with your legs stretched out in front of you. (If this is difficult, sit with your back against the wall.) Take a towel and sling it around your foot, across the ball of the foot, and pull the forefoot up toward you. You should feel a stretch in your calves and up behind the knees. Hold for 60 seconds.

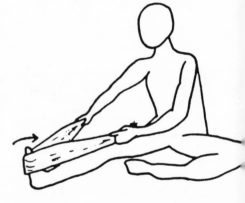

2. Hamstring Stretch—Sitting as in the first exercise, lean forward, place your hands on your calves and slide them down toward your toes, keep your knees straight. You should feel a stretch under your thighs. Try to keep your back relatively straight. Hold for 60 seconds.

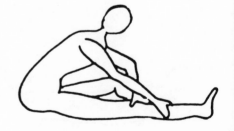

3. Butterfly Sit—Sit on the bed, floor or mat with your knees and hips bent. The soles of the feet touching. Clasp your ankles with your hands so that your elbows rest on the inside of your knees. Push the knees apart with your elbows as you lean forward. Hold for 60 seconds.

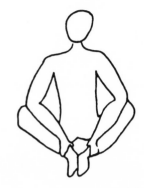

4. Wall Stretch—Lie on your back at the base of a wall—perpendicular to it (either on the floor or on a bed if it's against the wall). Your buttocks should be all the way up against the wall and your legs stretched out and up against the wall. Let the legs slowly separate and slide out to the side as far as possible. Hold for 60 seconds.

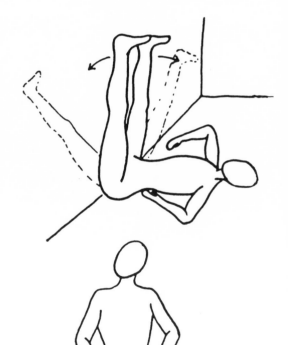

5. Kneel Standing—Get your knees on a mat or the floor. Then lower your buttocks down to the right heel and come back up. Then down to the left heel and back up again. Repeat 5-7 times—progress as tolerated.

Index

ACTH, 7
Allergen-free diet, 39
Amantidine, see Symmetrel
Ankle-foot orthosis, in the
    management of food drop, 29
Antidepressants, 93
Antivert, in the management of
    vertigo, 77
Atarax, in the management of
    tremor, 18
Autoimmune disease, 5
Autonomic nervous system, 4
Azathiaprine, see Imuran

Baclofen, see Lioresal
Benadryl, in the management of
    vertigo, 77
Benzoin, in the management of
    pressure sores, 81
Braces, in the management of foot
    drop, 29
Bracing, in the management of
    tremor, 19
Brainstem, 2
Bulk formers, for the
    management of constipation,
    65

Cane, use of, 30
Carbamepazine, see Tegretol

Catheterization, intermittent self-,
    56; chronic, 57
Central nervous system, 2
Cerebellum, 2; tremor from
    demyelination in, 18
Cerebrum, 2
Chronulac syrup, in the
    management of constipation,
    66
Clinitron bed, 82
Colace, in the management of
    constipation, 66
Constipation, 63
Contractures, 16
Corticosteroids, treatment with, 7
Crede technique, for bladder
    emptying, 56
Cyclobenzaprine HCl, see Flexoril
Cyclophosphamide, see Cytoxan
Cylert, for management of
    fatigue, 24
Cystospaz, in the management of
    bladder problems, 56
Cytoxan, 8

Dantrium, as anti-spasticity
    agent, 15
Debridement, in the management
    of pressure sores, 82

Notes

Notes

Notes

Notes

Notes

Notes